GRUMPY OLD MEN:
THE SECRET DIARY

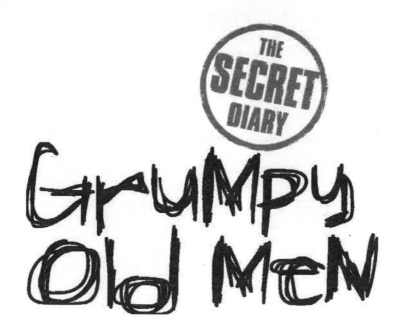

THE SECRET DIARY

GRUMPY OLD MEN

STUART PREBBLE

BBC
BOOKS

This book is published to accompany the television series *Grumpy Old Men*, first broadcast in 2003 (first series), 2004 (second series) and 2005 (third series). The series were produced by Liberty Bell Productions for BBC Television. Producer/Director: Stuart Prebble

First published in 2005
This edition published in 2007 by BBC Books, an imprint of Ebury Publishing

10 9 8 7 6 5 4 3 2

Ebury Publishing is a division of the Random House Group Ltd.

The Random House Group Ltd Reg. No. 954009

Addresses for companies within the Random House Group Ltd can be found at www.randomhouse.co.uk

A CIP catalogue record for this book is available from the British Library.

The Random House Group Ltd makes every effort to ensure that the papers used in our books are made from trees that have been legally sourced from well-managed and credibly certified forests. Our paper procurement policy can be found at www.randomhouse.co.uk

Commissioning editors: Shirley Patton and Stuart Cooper
Project editor: Sarah Reece Copy editor: Patricia Burgess
Designer: Linda Blakemore Illustrator: Noel Ford
Production: David Brimble

Set in Stone Serif and Erazure
Printed and bound in Great Britain by Cox & Wyman, Reading

ISBN 978 0 563 53923 0

Contents

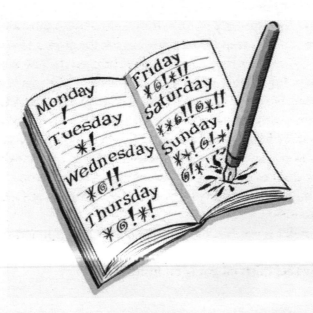

Introduction

I THOUGHT IT WAS JUST ME

I thought I was the only one who was walking or cycling or driving around gently shaking my head about just about everything I see or hear in the modern world. Just me with the little voice constantly going on inside my head, providing a running commentary on all the little niggles and irritations and nonsenses and preposterous, patent absurdities that seem to have been dreamt up with the specific intention of getting on my nerve endings.

I am a fully grown-up adult, have held down a job, brought up a family, taken responsibility for myself for quite a few years now; yet someone somewhere has just changed the law to stop me from doing some simple electrical wiring in my own house. In my long-ago hippy days, I hitch-hiked halfway around the world, but now someone else gets to decide that I have to wear a seat-belt if I sit in the back of a car. I've been taking the same route to work day in day out for years and years, and one day someone decides to block off two lanes, prevent me from turning right at my usual junction, and to charge me £5 a day for the privilege.

I thought it was just me gently seething and simmering. Occasionally mouthing some vile expletive or other, but generally keeping it all going on inside.

Then along came *Grumpy Old Men*; and when I interviewed a whole selection of blokes of a certain age and a certain temperament, it turned out that exactly the same stuff that pisses me off pisses them off in equal measure – sometimes even more.

Well, it was bad enough when I thought it was just me. Since no one has been taking a blind bit of notice of anything I've said for years, I hadn't expected anyone to take any notice of me now. I'd reluctantly seethe in silence as the train conductor told me the same information on entering every station, once in every station, and having just left every station on the six-hour journey that should have lasted for three. I'd just put up with patronizing 12-year-olds in electrical appliance shops talking to me as though I was their geriatric uncle.

But now I know it's not just me. Since the series went out, I've discovered that just about everybody – everybody with any sense, that is – thinks that the world has gone bloody mad. So now that we know it's damned nearly all of us, we're wondering why we have to tolerate it. If, as it seems to turn out, most of us think the world has been taken over by arse-heads whose sole purpose in life is to irritate us, why do we all have to put up with it?

What started out as an individual affliction has become something of a source of strength. Where once there might have been some potential embarrassment at adopting the label of 'Grumpy Old Man', now it has become a badge of honour. We know that we're not alone and, yes, we are as mad as hell and we ain't gonna take it any more.

Recently we have welcomed some distinguished names into our fold. Founding members, such as Arthur Smith, Rory McGrath, Will Self, Rick Wakeman and John O'Farrell, have been joined by self-confessed grumpies, such as John Stapleton, Don Warrington, Des Lynam, Nigel Havers and Sir Gerry Robinson.

And what their various testimonies confirm is that grumpiness is not an occasional mood or a temporary feeling. Not a personality disorder or a treatable condition. It's a way of looking at the world. Everyday life for those of us of a grumpy persuasion is nothing but a series of irritants and obstacles, most of them deliberately put in our way by jackasses. Every single day it's the same old things – or rather it's a mix of the same old things, and a lot of new things that the nothing-if-not-inventive boneheads come up with to add to our grumpidom.

So when I told the BBC this, and that I was going to chronicle it for a new book and a third series, they said that I must be exaggerating. Even I, with my now legendarily low tolerance levels, couldn't come up with some new irritation for every day of the year.

Well, of course I haven't come up with a new grump for every day of the year. I could – oh, believe me I could – but to do so would risk irritating myself and you even further. However, what I think I have done is to show how grumpiness spreads pretty evenly right across the year. It is impervious to seasons, national holidays, special occasions, trips abroad … It just is.

So this is a diary. And what's secret about it? Well, there's nothing secret about it. You just bought it, for Christ's sake. The plain fact is that we just thought you'd be more likely to buy it with 'secret' in the title. There; that's something to get you in the right mood …

STUART PREBBLE

January

1 JANUARY

When you are young and you hear older people use expressions such as 'I feel as though I've been hit by a truck,' you think it's just a fairly meaningless figure of speech, don't you? Just some old git exaggerating. That's if you even pause for a moment to listen to or care what he's talking about, which probably you don't.

But when struggling to think of a description that conveys my state this morning, only one comes close to accurately indicating what I actually feel. 'I feel as though I've been hit by a truck.'

My body aches – right from the very hard shell at the top of my cranium to the hard skin on the soles of my feet that usually feels as though it must belong to somebody else. Top to toe and every cubic inch in between, as though every cell is reacting to some physical trauma, like a car crash. Every muscle hurting; every joint jarred and bruised to buggery.

I woke up at 9 a.m., which is about four hours later than I usually do, but still three hours earlier than I would like to have done, sprawled and prone like one of those cartoon characters that has been flattened and has to peel itself off the pavement. I'm stuck to the bed, the slightest movement producing only a more excruciating twinge of pain.

Don't sit there feeling holier than I, because you've done this. Yes, you have. Be honest. Let he who is without sin cast the first stone. You lie there with your eyes closed, trying to remain inside your own head as long as possible, before even considering attempting to come to terms with the world you've woken up in. You may emit a small groan, but find that it doesn't help. At all.

Unwelcome images swim uncontrollably around your head; memories of the previous night. The sea of faces, their expressions betraying ever greater alcohol-induced delirium, going on and on and on and on about what a crap year it's been. And all you can think of is 'What the fuck is this idiot talking about?' or 'When on earth will he pause long enough so I can go and find someone, anyone, less terminally stupid to talk to?' Then, in what will ultimately prove to be a futile effort to numb the pain, you hear yourself utter those dreadful words, 'Oh, go on then, what the hell, it's only once a year.'

Why does it always have to be this way? After every celebration of any kind, large or small, even when you've started out with the very best intentions of keeping everything in moderation, not eating or drinking anything really stupid or in copious amounts, even then, you wake up feeling like the proverbial rat's gizzard that's been extruded through a sausage-making machine. Why?

Now I want to report fairly quickly that my head was not surrounded on all sides by dried vomit, as at one time it might have been on 1 January. No, unfortunately or otherwise, those days are long behind me, and the idea that I should attend a party that would end with such consequences is far back in history. In those days I would drink eight pints of draught Guinness in the course of an evening, stagger back to my bed, and then live through that dreadful and totally disconcerting ordeal of spinning in outer space every time I closed my eyes.

Did this happen to you? It must have. You'd close them for a few moments, hoping to go off to sleep, but your entire body would feel as though it was literally going into rotation – like

you were on an out-of-control space-walk – and would continue
to spin at a fast-increasing velocity until you opened your eyes
and struggled to regain your bearings. Then you'd have another
go, closing your eyes and hoping to lose consciousness before
the spinning became unbearable, but usually having to pull
yourself around a few times. Eventually, you would lose
consciousness and disappear into a black hole.

On the worst of these occasions, you'd be vaguely aware
during the night of having to get up a couple of times to throw
up; and yes, let's admit it, on the very worst occasions you'd
wake up in the morning having failed to make it. Oh, groo. In
the morning you'd rush to the lavatory, retch the remaining
lining from your stomach and a few bits of carrot – even
though you haven't eaten carrot for three days. Then you'd
press your head against the cooling porcelain, gently mouthing
the words, 'Never again, never again'. Poetic isn't it? Almost
Edgar Allan Poe.

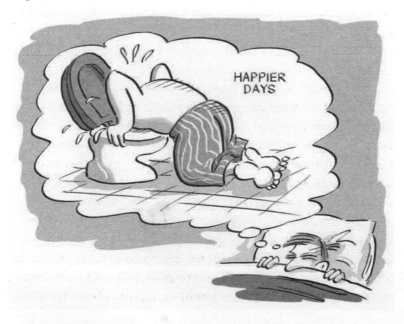

But that was all a long time ago, and the sad thing is that the blurred memories of wild new year's eve parties, which were just that – blurred – by excessive alcohol and revelry, are long since things of the past. These days we are all far too sad and grumpy even to try to recapture such times.

Some years my wife and I talk about having a '60s party' to which all our friends will come, wearing what they got married in, or what they wore to the Isle of Wight festival in 1969. We'll drink loads of cheap wine, burn some incense sticks, play loads of Hendrix and Cream, and maybe someone will even bring some grass.

Leaving aside the obvious hindrance that few, if any, of our friends could locate such outfits, and if they could, they certainly wouldn't be able to squeeze their spreading frames into them, what makes such an event less plausible is that no one would really be 'up for it'.

What it seems we all are 'up for', if anything, is a rather civilized gathering at someone's house, where moderate amounts of alcohol will be served with moderate amounts of hors d'oeuvres, while we all chit-chat about what a bloody awful year it's been. Then, when midnight is approaching, we put the telly on and flick the channels between Jools Holland's programme (which lost its appeal for me when someone pointed out that it had obviously been pre-recorded some time earlier), and some twot of a Scotsman playing bagpipes at what looks and sounds like a very forced form of revelry.

At midnight we wish each other a happy new year, kiss one another on the cheeks rather awkwardly, shake hands even more awkwardly with the blokes, and wonder whether we can now slip away. Out in the street we forget which one of us has agreed to drink in moderation and, because my wife has always drunk less than me, she ends up braving what seems like the bloody dodgems in the hope of getting us home in one piece.

Yes, that's what they're like, the new year's eve celebrations of a Grumpy Old Man. Exhilarating, isn't it?

So anyway, you'd think that the one redeeming feature of all this utter bollocks would be that you'd wake up feeling fine and refreshed. But not a bit of it. You feel as though you've been hit by a truck, and that's because you've stood in more or less one place for five bloody hours, sipped what probably added up to a bottle of wine and eaten a lot of gourmet cocktail sausages. Dipped in mustard.

What could be less fair than waking up feeling dreadful after an evening like that? Fair enough if you'd done the eight pints, spent the night carousing on the dancefloor and taken a lunge at a policeman on the way home. But no, not a bit of it. This is how I now feel after even a moderate celebration.

This is what it's come to. I think a quiet rest of day is called for, don't you?

2 JANUARY

Of course, I'm thinking all this stuff because it's January, and I'm grumpy. Grumpy all the time these days, about everything, but my grumpiness takes on a particular flavour at this time of the year. Christmas is over, thank God, for another year, and I keep hearing people talk about their 'new year resolutions'.

Actually, what I hear people talking about is their 'new year's resolutions', as though the resolutions belong to the year rather than to them, but that's just a trivial piece of torment that even I usually manage to stop myself from pointing out. One can get a bit boring, I fear.

According to the original survey that spawned the 'Grumpy Old Man' phenomenon (if I may call it that), men aged 35–54 are the grumpiest group in history. Grumpier than their parents, who survived the war and mostly went on to draw their pensions and move to Lanzarote or Alicante, where they spent, or are spending, their children's inheritance and their own last years watching Sky Sports and playing bingo or whatever they do, in somewhere called the King's Head. Grumpier than their children, who seem to be getting on with their lives and suffering far less angst about the state of the world we have left them with than we might expect or that we would have felt ourselves.

No, this is the group that, when asked a series of questions designed to find out how happy and optimistic it is, tends to give the most negative answers.

Do we think the world is becoming a safer place? Hell, no. Sure, we were the generation who lived through the Cuban missile crisis, but at least in those days we believed that the enemy wanted to stay alive as much as we did. We called it 'mutually assured destruction', which, in the 1960s, was thought to be a deterrent. Seems like our enemies today would regard that as a fast ticket to paradise.

Or do we think our old age will be as comfortable as that of our parents? Of course not – most of those who survived went into jobs for life, and got to retirement age before index-linked pensions became a thing of the past for all but a few judges and politicians.

No, we're the ones most irritated by all the 'stuff' that gets in our way or up one of our orifices (orifi?) on a daily basis – mobile phones with the ringtone of a horse whinnying, an apparently endless stream of cloned politicians talking to us as though we're mentally challenged, overcrowded trains, boats and planes that never, simply never, run on time. In short, we're the ones least likely to think the world is becoming a better place, and it eludes us how any rational person could look at it and think otherwise

So anyway, to cut a long story short (which people often

announce as their intention but seldom actually do), I'm 53.
According to the statistics and the half-arsed theory, I should
be emerging out of this most grumpy phase; and may be
metamorphosing into what should be the more mellow, more
accepting time of my life.

That's partly the point of keeping this diary – to see if I do,
and if I do, perhaps thereby to offer some hope to all those
among you who identify with the 'Grumpy Old Man' syndrome
(maybe 'syndrome' is better than 'phenomenon' – sounds
more like an affliction and ever so slightly less like a piece of
pretentious shite). Also, and more particularly, to offer solace
to their wives and their loved ones. Because one thing for
certain is that my wife and family sure as hell are hoping that
I'm shortly going to be getting more mellow. The trouble is, on
all the available evidence recently, I'm just getting a whole hell
of a lot worse.

3 JANUARY

The world is full of electronic bleeping. It's everywhere. Our
lives are ruled by it.

Bleeping when you set the microwave or unlock the car.
Bleeping when you fail to fasten your safety belt or are running
out of windscreen wash. Bleeping when you send a text or set
the house alarm. Hundreds and hundreds of bloody bleeps
when you go through the supermarket checkout, and bleeping
at 100 decibels if the shopkeeper has failed to deactivate the
bar-code on the DVD or T-shirt you just bought.

I mention it because today I was so busy looking for my
mobile phone that I was nearly knocked over by the dustcart
that was reversing towards me. Made a note to change the
ringtone.

4 JANUARY

Yes, this truly is a depressing time of the year, isn't it? That's probably why new year resolutions were invented. Something to give us the brief delusion that this year the world won't be quite as crap as last year. It's obviously a totally ridiculous notion that some artificial moment in a calendar can help us to make our lives better. But because we're all idiots, quite a few of us fall for it.

Left to myself, I'd certainly ignore them. I guess I assume that the world would be a far better place if other people adjusted their behaviour to be more like mine rather than the other way around. However, this season usually cannot be allowed to pass by without someone in the family suggesting that I should amend a couple of things.

'What?' I ask, already indicating that I'm very unlikely to embrace the suggestion with much of a sense of celebration.

'How about "Must try harder to form some kind of relationship with Matt?"' (my 17-year-old son) is my wife's suggestion this year. As, indeed, I seem to recall it was last year, and probably even the year before. Why? When I was 17 I wanted a 'relationship' with my father about as desperately as I wanted a dose of the clap. Few things were lower down my list of priorities. Why should it be any different today?

Well, of course, the answer should be that, unlike my dad, I am a child of the '60s. Whereas he grew up during the Great Depression, fought in the war, and believed that if your hair touched the top of your ears or your collar you were a poofter, I grew up at the dawning of the Age of Aquarius. I am cool, easy-going, tolerant and nowhere near as bigoted and unreasonable as my dad was at this stage in our respective lives. What, therefore, could my son possibly have to rebel against? The answer, of course, is that he doesn't rebel – it's so much worse than that –

he doesn't seem to do anything. Which drives me crazy. And I show it. So he ignores me. Which drives me crazier still. So it might be preferable if we had a better relationship. Which just irritates me more.

Then there's Lizzie, our 15-year-old daughter. With her I find it much easier to identify an area to try to resolve. 'Must find a way to make her stop choosing her boyfriends purely on the basis of how extremely they're going to irritate me.' I know that seems a bit egocentric, imagining that she cares enough what her mother or I think about anything for it to influence her in either direction; but in this case I really think there's something in it.

Of the dozen or so boyfriends of one kind or another she's had in the last eighteen months since she started 'dating', only one looks as though he didn't arrive directly from a sewer, and I made the patently ridiculous mistake of saying something mildly complimentary about him. Needless to say, he didn't last the weekend. Every one since then has been a variation of ghastly: we've had the purple-haired Mohican without piercings; we've had the one with no hair at all but with piercings; we've had dreadlocks without piercings but with tattoos; we've had floppy hair with and without safety pins; we had one who seemed to think it was OK for at least 50 per cent of his pimply arse to be on show, and another whose crotch was so low that he looked like a fucking tadpole. And not one of them was able to answer any question with anything more articulate than a grunt.

I'd be the first to admit that I was never going to be easy to please in this matter. When Lizzie was growing up, before she became as bad-tempered as a very bad-tempered person who's just been jabbed by an electronic cattle-prod, I used to try to set some standards for anyone wishing to become my future son-in-law.

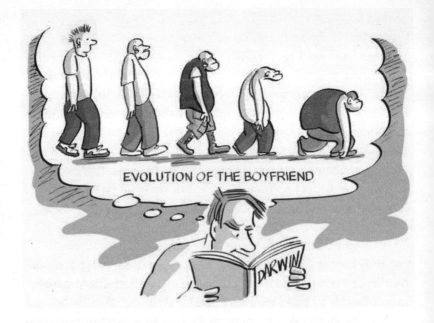

EVOLUTION OF THE BOYFRIEND

'I don't care if his surname is Gates, and he's the more talented middle brother between Bill and Gareth, he still won't be good enough for you,' I used to quip, hilariously.

The latest, whose name I've been unable yet to commit to memory, but sounds like Vader or Vaguer, does not quite get over this bar. Truth to tell, he is a combination of all the worst features of his predecessors, and, just to make my life complete, is unemployed. And Polish. Needless to say, I recently made the mistake of suggesting to Lizzie that maybe she could do a bit better, at which point she started talking about feeling that it was time she made a commitment.

'She's just saying that to scare you,' says my wife.

'Well, it's working.' This is a hard one, which I know is going to tax us heavily in the year ahead.

5 JANUARY

Sitting in the kitchen this morning and becoming ever more irritated by our cats. Brother and sister, they're ten years old, and still neither of them has worked out that the furry thing that moves about at the edge of their peripheral vision is their tail. I suppose that some people can find stupidity in an animal endearing for a period, but ten years?

These animals eat too much, leave fur all over the place, scratch the carpets and wallpaper, puke up in the middle of the floor, crap in the litter tray rather than in someone else's garden, and catch and disembowel defenceless creatures. They're also stupid.

Maybe you can understand why one of them can't work out that its tail is attached, but you'd think the other might have mentioned it by now, wouldn't you?

I keep on asking – as innocently as I can – what ten cat years equal in human years. Unfortunately, the family knows what this is code for, and simply assures me that they can easily live at least another five years. So the little buggers will probably outlive me.

8 JANUARY

The best joke of all at this time of year, of course, is the number of people who say 'This is the year in which I'm going to get fit.' I know this well because, of course, I've done it.

What a laugh.

In January every year, year in year out, attendance at the local gym is at a 12-month high. We have allowed ourselves to put on a few extra pounds in the run-up to Christmas because, let's face it, the weather was dark and depressing, and anyway we could wear more clothes, which enabled us to disguise those hideous bulges that wallowed and splurged over our belts when we sat down.

Then we were coming up to Christmas, when we knew there was a good chance that we'd pig out, so what was the point of watching our diets too ferociously just now? Then came Christmas itself and, despite our good intentions not to 'go mad' this year, we did.

Well, maybe not mad exactly, but certainly slightly disturbed.

Too much turkey, even though it was dry and god-awful and gave us constipation. Too much Christmas pudding or too many mince pies. Too many chocolate brazils or Quality Street or, heaven help us, too much crystallized fruit. What on earth is that about? And, of course, far too much alcohol.

We're disgusted with ourselves and we all say – never mind, first thing in the new year I'm going on a diet. And we join the gym.

If all the people who sign up for the gym in January actually attended, every gymnasium in the land would be massively over-subscribed and have to expand faster than your waistline in December, or close down. But neither of these prospects detains them for a minute because they know us better than we know ourselves.

They know that we're going to wince at the 30- or 40- or 50-quid-a-month membership fee – which is usually paid a year up front for reasons we're about to see – and console ourselves by saying, 'Well, I'm paying all that money, so at least it means it'll force me to go.' The trouble is that you also think that by merely joining the gym you've done the work. Or the hard bit at least. You almost expect to start shedding the pounds as soon as you've signed the bank mandate. Of course, you know what's coming next – you *are* shedding pounds – it's just that they're in sterling rather than imperial. Certainly the stress of parting with all that money brings on so much anxiety for me that I'd expect to lose half a stone in a couple of hours.

What happens is that you go once or twice, or three times, or maybe as much as half a dozen; you marvel at how totally unfit you are; you damn nearly give yourself a heart attack by overdoing it in the first few sessions; you get on the scales before and after every session of exercise and find that they haven't budged a millimetre. Or if they have, it may even be in altogether the wrong direction.

And that's because exercise doesn't make you lose weight. Not really. It's a popular myth, I know, but take it from me, it just doesn't. Recently I saw a statistic on a poster that was part of the BBC's humiliating and patronizing *Fat Nation* campaign that asked, 'Did you know that if you run a mile three times a week, you'll lose 12 lb over the course of a year?'

What? So in the wholly implausible event that I could summon the energy to put on my shorts, T-shirt, socks and running shoes, and go out on to the busy High Street and run a mile three times a week for a year, I'd lose only 12 lb? When I saw that I said to the person I was with that if I was running the campaign (an unlikely eventuality, but far more likely than that I would be running the miles), I'd keep that particular statistic a secret.

All that effort and you wouldn't even lose a stone? A mile, three times a week every week for 52 weeks in a row, and you'd lose only two inches round your gut?

No, I'm afraid that exercise doesn't make you lose weight. If you take a trip on any of those exercise machines that monitor various aspects of your performance as you ski up mountains or row down rapids or whatever it is, the calorie counter goes up very, very slowly, and you find that after half an hour of blood, sweat and tears, you might have lost about 500 calories. Well, that's hardly the equivalent of a slice of pizza. You are totally, utterly drained and knackered to the extent that you can hardly raise your leg to step into the bath, and all you've earned is the right to a Mars bar. Scarcely even that.

So why, if I think it's all so much bollocks, have I fallen for it again this year? Basically because I'm 54 at the end of this year and am sick to death of waking up in the morning and feeling like I'm 84. If I don't get myself moving on a regular basis now, I never will. So I've signed the banker's order form, made the personal commitment to go once or twice a week and yes, quite literally, got the T-shirt with 'Piss-Pots Gym', or whatever it is, written on the front. And do you know what? When they asked me what size I needed, I said 'large', when the truth is that I'm more comfortable in an 'extra large'. Yes, I'm deluding myself that after half a dozen visits, 'large' will fit me perfectly well.

11 JANUARY

Don't you just hate it when politicians go on the telly and say the same thing over and over again? We've just had that very strange woman Ruth Kelly on the box. Although she looks more like the head girl than one of the teachers, we're asked to believe that she's now the Education Secretary, and she was on about 'working with teachers to develop a common-sense approach to school trips'. Then she was asked another question, and she said that this illustrated exactly the sort of problem that made her want to 'work closely with teachers to develop a common-sense approach towards school trips'. Then something else, and her reply was about how keen she was to sit down with teachers to work out an agreed approach towards school trips. OK, we got that, anything else to say? No? Well, get off then.

Gordon Brown does that. Listen to him next time. He's got one thing to say, and whatever the interviewer asks him, he goes on saying that same thing over and over. Drives you bonkers.

12 JANUARY

Back to work today. Oh joy, oh bliss, oh shit. I managed to leave it for as long as possible, but inevitably the day arrives.

It's not that I have anything much against work itself. Once I'm in the office, I can find it a welcome diversion from most of the things that irritate me when I've been hanging around the house for too long – and certainly it's a relief for the family. It's everything else.

At the weekends and when I've got nothing particular to do, I always wake up well before dawn and am soon fidgeting and have to get out of bed. On the rare occasions that I could stay in bed longer, it's always a day when I have to get up and go to work. Do you find that?

I look in the mirror, feel depressed, wonder if I need to shave, and look in my diary to see if I have to meet someone who'll gave a damn if I've shaved or not. Mostly there's one person who I know will look down their nose at me if I'm sporting what could be misinterpreted as 'designer stubble' when in reality it's 'designer idleness', so I do.

If it's cold and I'm feeling mawkish, I use an old electric razor, which is so old and close to useless that the other day it actually cut the side of my mouth. The upside is that it is less of a shock to the system early in the morning than a wet shave; the downside is that my eyesight and general carelessness is now at a level when I often find that I've missed parts of my face.

I'll be sitting in a meeting later in the day stroking my chin or touching my filtrum, when I'll feel a little area of bristle that I've overlooked. Usually just under a nostril or next to an ear.

Now even I know that this is as clear and unambiguous a sign of old-gitdom as you'll ever experience. I remember as a kid occasionally chortling with my brother that my grandad had left an isolated area of stubble on his face, like a desert island sprouting palm trees. Not only do I do this myself now, but I do it regularly. I keep resolving that I should carry a little disposable razor in my pocket or case so that I can nip off to the men's room and deal with these things when they arise. But, of course, even that would be too late. By then everyone in the office has no doubt noticed and chortled at the senile old fart, just as my brother and I did 45 years ago with our poor old grandad. They say everything that goes around comes around, and it does.

Then I have to decide whether to shower or bath. I find I alternate between the two, depending on the weather and how fat and stiff I'm feeling. When it's cold or I'm feeling unusually fat or I've been exerting myself in some small way and feel stiff, I prefer the bath. Either is a bloody nuisance. I used to get real pleasure out of a bath or a shower. Now it's just getting wet.

Then the vexatious decision about what to wear. I know I'm lucky these days not to have a proper job and not to need to wear a suit to work, but I still find that I cultivate a uniform. I have five pairs of black 501s on the go at any one time, and occasionally it occurs to me that loads of people must think I wear the same pair every day. I care about this, but apparently

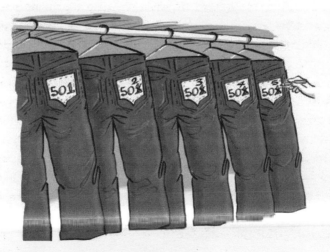

not enough to buy even slightly different trousers. I have about ten black or dark blue soft-collared shirts from Marks & Spencer, and four more or less identical blue pullovers.

Then there's the haircut. Basically all my life I've detested going to get my hair cut, and so has every grumpy I know. As a kid you always had to get a 'short back and sides' and you'd come out with the proverbial pudding-basin style and your young and tender neck red raw. Thanks, Ron.

There were all those years when you thought your hair was a key factor in whether or not you were going to get laid, and the hairdresser always, always managed to make you look even more of a dork than nature intended. I'd give the barber strict instructions not to cut it too high off my collar or above my ears, and I'd always come out bloody mortified, to the extent that I felt sure that everyone in the street was looking at me and thinking 'What a prat'. I'm still by no means convinced that they were not.

Then you could never persuade the barber that you didn't want 'something on it' or that you didn't want to leave the shop with hair like someone from a sodding menswear catalogue and so you'd have to muss it up the minute you got into the street.

Anyway, it's been variations on this theme for the 40 years since. Hours of queuing in depressing 'salons', being overcharged, and coming out looking like a refugee from 'Lord Snooty and His Pals'. So a few years ago I bought my own electric razor from Boots, and now, every time I get fed up, I set it to number five, put a towel round my shoulders and run it over my own head. I know I look like one of those kids who used to come to your primary school from the orphanage, but frankly I'm past caring.

So that's me. I look the same every day of the week. A blotchy shave, the haircut from hell, more or less the same clothes, the net result looking as much as anything like a sort of obese scarecrow. A triumph of indolence over vanity.

And do you know what? When I met most of the original cast of *Grumpy Old Men* – Arthur, Rory, Will Self, Ken Stott, et al – they all looked more or less the same. Matthew Parris takes the thing to an extreme – he looks as though he's slept on a park bench. A pitiful sight we all are, no doubt, but hey – who gives a damn? We're old, we're grumpy and we don't give a toss.

'My hairdresser actually spends more time now digging hair out of my ears than off the top or the back of my head. She has got this little thing that buzzes in and out of my ears. Then I got home the other day and I found there were actually hairs growing not so much in my ear, but on the top of my ear. I thought it was hair from my head. It's actually growing round the rim of my ear. What's that all about? I don't need my ears to be protected in that way by hair. It's a design fault, an absolute design fault.'

DES LYNAM

13 JANUARY

Saw the first Easter egg in the shops today. Three months away from Easter, a carton full of Cadbury's Creme Eggs on the counter at the garage. Right under your nose when you pay for your petrol. Three hundred million Easter eggs sold in Britain every year; six each for every man, woman and child in the country. No wonder they have to start early.

Planned to go to Piss-Pots this evening for my first workout under my rigorous new regime, but felt too knackered, so decided to start in earnest next week.

14 JANUARY

How did I get to have a daughter doing maths at A level?
Sometimes I really think there must have been a mix-up in the
hospital and we took home the wrong kid. I used to quite like it
when she'd come home and want a bit of help with history or
English, or even geography, because there was a fair chance I
might be able to show off by knowing the capital of France or
the main industry in the Ruhr. I remember her struggling one
day with her French homework, and being amazed that her
father appeared to be able to speak a bit of French. Tonight she
asked me what logarithms were actually for. It's a question I
recall asking myself a lot when I was 17 and had failed my
maths O level twice. I don't seem to recall having had to answer
it much since.

'You're hopeless,' she said, and in that respect, at least, I could
do nothing but agree.

15 JANUARY

The sales – and I can almost hear you asking why someone as
terminally grumpy as I am would dream of going shopping
during the January sales. Well, the clue lies in the fact that next
to my grumpiness my most endearing feature is my meanness.

And funnily enough, by this point in the calendar, the sales
are nowhere near as horrendous as you might think. They've
been on for about three weeks and are more or less over, and
everything has been pawed by thousands of grasping and
groping hands, and the only things left are the total rejects that
nobody else wants. The crowds have therefore dwindled to a
trickle of sad ne'er-do-wells, such as myself, who don't really
care what they look like as long as they don't have to pay the
full price.

These few days are the only time of the year when a combination of my basic needs pertains: the prices are about 40 per cent of their usual level – which means that in a few cases you are paying a sum close to what something is actually worth, and there are not hordes of people about.

This is when I do my clothes shopping for the whole of the coming year. I buy two pairs of casual shoes, two pairs of black Levis, a pair of chinos, a couple of sweatshirts, a couple of T-shirts, a pullover and that's me done. All in about an hour and a half.

I usually briefly toy with the idea of buying a bomber or leather jacket that is far too young for me; it's been reduced from £400 to £200, but still, in the end, I balk at the price. Which means I'm back at home in time for elevenses.

Now that's what I call shopping – assuming that you have to do any at all. I guess I'm really looking forward to the day when I need to care so little about what anyone thinks of the way I look that I don't actually need to go shopping at all. I'll look at my last couple of pairs of 501s and say 'Well, they'll see me out.' Maybe that's part of the process of getting more mellow as you get older. Less stuff to piss you off.

17 JANUARY

There was an item on the news today about how, during a press conference in Spain, David Beckham spoke a sentence in Spanish.

That's right; after, I think, two years of living in Spain, extensive Spanish lessons with the best teachers that money can buy, and working almost exclusively in a Spanish-speaking environment, David Beckham managed to speak a single sentence in halting Spanish. Even so, I gather that the grammar was questionable.

And this event is deemed important enough to make the national news on British television. Since I just don't know where to start, I won't.

'I think Gary Lineker set the example. And then Paul Gascoigne spent a couple of years in Italy and learnt the word "pizza", which was very good. And now David Beckham has mastered the Spanish language and comes out with the odd word – "paella", for example. No, David Beckham speaking Spanish, very impressive; maybe English will be next.'

JOHN O'FARRELL

19 JANUARY

All the advertisements on the telly are for holidays. Florida, Greece, Tunisia, Spain. Pictures of bronzed and smiling families frolicking in the surf. This always causes a bit of tension in our house because I'm well known to hate holidays, and by and large would prefer to stay at home. Somehow or other, though, it seems obvious that we've got to go on one.

Over the years I've tried various tactics, from delay – 'Let's wait and see what bargains we can get closer to the time' – to generalized negativity – 'Bloke at work went there and had a terrible time.' I've decided that my tactic this year is to be indecision – today I said, 'Maybe it would be nice to drive down the coast from New York to Carolina?' But then next time the subject comes up I'll say, 'Maybe we should just tour the West Country and stay in some B&Bs.'

Will be sure to record how we get on.

22 JANUARY

Yes, I know, I know, already I've been missing a few days, but keeping a diary was never my best thing. Did you do this as a kid? Sometimes your auntie or your grandma would buy you a diary for Christmas. You'd try to express enthusiasm, then put it aside and get on playing with your blow-football, spinning-top, or 'compendium of games', including snakes and ladders and draughts.

After a few days and a few tears caused by fighting with your brother, you'd be so bored that you'd spend a couple of hours writing your name and address and the names of your friends and even your hobbies in the front of the diary. You'd write a little entry every day – 'Got up, played chess, had cheese on toast for tea, watched *The Cisco Kid*, went to bed' – for about four days – maybe rediscover it briefly in April and write a bit more, and that was it for the year.

Well, I'm going to do better than that this time. Dunno how much better, but the thing to remember is that there'll be no point in counting the days. Sure, there's stuff that makes Grumpy Old Men grumpy every single day of the year. More than enough. It's just that sometimes we're too grumpy to write it down.

25 JANUARY

As we're nearly at the end of the first month, this may be a good time to pause for a moment for newcomers to the idea and consider the condition of the Grumpy Old Man.

The first thing to understand about the Grumpy Old Man is that usually he is not grumpy in the sense of being miserable or even generally unhappy. When we were making the first TV series, we asked all sorts of people to participate, some of whom were quite offended at the notion that they might be perceived as falling into the category.

For example, I wanted to ask Lenny Henry, but his agent told me that Lenny is the most irredeemably cheerful person that he knows. I had to point out that this does not disqualify him. Grumpy Old Men are not necessarily that grumpy; they are people who simply cannot stop themselves from seeing the preposterous everywhere they look. And often pointing it out.

Would you like a very simple test of this? OK, here goes; today my wife and I were sitting in a traffic jam listening to the news on the radio. I wasn't really concentrating, but I caught the words 'every six seconds someone calls the Samaritans'.

I know that a normal person would react by saying something like 'That's awful,' or even, 'Maybe we should volunteer.' However, I just couldn't stop myself saying, 'Christ, I bet they wish he'd just stay on the line and finish the sodding phone call.' Idiotic, I know, but I just can't help it – and nor can any other Grumpy Old Man. It's the cross we have to bear.

The next thing is that Grumpy Old Men are not necessarily old. I've been amazed to discover over the past couple of years that the tortured state of mind I'm talking about seems to be almost as common among 25-year-olds as it is among 35- or 45-year-olds. And my new friend Geoffrey Palmer, who enjoys the series so much that he's started moving his holidays around so that he can record the commentary, says he recognizes everything in it. Geoffrey (I hope he won't mind me telling you) is older than 55.

And, of course, the last thing is that Grumpy Old Men don't have to be men. Indeed, my excellent colleague Judith Holder has admirably pointed out the teaming mass of stuff that gets on the wick of her fellow Grumpy Old Women. Yes, much of it is the same as ours – kids, people serving in shops, and all the debris and detritus of getting old. The main difference is, of course, that women think it's OK to go on at great length about what's wrong with men, whereas we know better. We might think the same about women but … Well, let's just say that we know better.

So, Grumpy Old Men – not necessarily grumpy, not necessarily old and not necessarily men. Anything you can identify with here?

'Grumpiness is reality. It's the fact that you know so many things are wrong. So many things are horrendous, from politics to health, to cars, to people. And there's nothing you can do about it. So the way to release that is just to be grumpy. You can moan and it gets it out of your system.'

RICK WAKEMAN

27 JANUARY

Is it just me, or does it get on your nerves when the weather forecasters tell you what to wear?

'There are going to be some chilly winds, so if you're going out, don't forget to wrap up nice and warm.'

This epitomizes much of what irritates me on the telly. What I want out of a weather forecaster is the weather forecast. I don't want to know what it's been like today. I've been alive today, and I know what it's been like. To be honest, I don't even want to know what it's going to be like at 2 a.m. or 4 a.m. All I want is some idea of what it's going to be like tomorrow and the next few days after that.

I've long since stopped believing the forecast, and I don't

plan to reiterate my theory that more often than not you'd be better off consulting a piece of seaweed, but if it really is inevitable that the skies are going to open later on this afternoon, it would be good to have a word of warning.

What I don't need, however, and what I venture to suggest that none of us needs, is some patronizing dildo-head telling us that we should wrap up nice and warm. You tell us the weather, we'll decide what to wear. OK?

28 JANUARY

Well, the forecaster's idea of 'chilly winds' turned out to be a blizzard, and today the weather went very quickly through the whole gamut from 'Aaah, isn't it pretty?' through 'Bloody hell, it had better stop in a minute,' to 'Shit, we can't get the car up the hill.' So, naturally enough, the whole bloody country has ground to a halt.

What amazes me is that it always seems to be a surprise. Like it never snows here, so we weren't expecting it, and straight away everything is chaos. Trains don't run, tubes get stuck in tunnels, miles and miles of lorries end up queuing to get to the ports, their drivers lighting fires underneath the engines – which I always thought must be jolly dangerous. Mountain rescue teams getting people out of the cars stuck in snowdrifts across the Pennines, and we're always treated to a description from the weather girl of her journey to work.

Let's face it, it's the same thing every bloody year. Why can't we stop being surprised?

29 JANUARY

A glance at my bank statement reminds me that I'm paying £40 a month to Piss-Pots for my gym membership and still haven't been. The evil angel on my shoulder advises me to face facts and cancel the standing order straight away, but then the good angel chastises me for my indolence and I resolve to go next week. All this struggling with difficult decisions is exhausting stuff.

February

2 FEBRUARY

At lunchtime today my wife called me at work and said we'd had a power cut. She was just defrosting the freezer – had all the stuff out and wrapped in freezer bags – and was chipping away at the ice like bloody Amundsen, when everything went off. So she had to put it all back in and close the door.

'Have you reported it?'

'I'm reporting it now.'

'How do you mean?'

'To you. I thought you might like to deal with it. I don't know, it seems like a "bloke thing".'

Obviously, I'd like to deal with it. Nothing I want to do more. Nothing better to do at work other than to sit and listen to some canned Vivaldi for an hour until some air-head fobs me off.

'OK, leave it to me,' I say, trying to strike a very fine balance so that she knows I'm inconvenienced, but hey, I'm the kind of guy who's willing to take on these things.

Obviously there is no such thing as a telephone directory any more, and equally obviously the relevant company is not called anything as simple as the 'Electricity Board' – and anyway, these days, for all I know, we get our electricity from the bakers. We certainly get our bread from the milkman, but that's another story.

Anyway, eventually, after about five calls to variations of 118 etc., I ascertain that it's called London Energy and, guess what, I'm answered by a long recorded menu of options.

'If you are calling from a push-button phone, press the hash key twice now.' Long pause while I try to find my glasses and the hash key. 'Now press 1 to pay your bill, press 2 for a meter reading, press 3 if you are moving house, press 4 for details of our charges, or wait for an operator.'

Then the music starts, and it's not Vivaldi. Today's it's the Ride of the Valkyries. I guess they must alternate. I wait. And wait. And every minute or so a voice comes on saying that my call is being held in a queue and an operator will be with me soon. They don't have a system that tells you where you are in the queue, so for all I know all the households in Kingston that are without electricity are in the queue. All 40,000 of them.

At the moment when I'm about to start eating my own flesh, a live voice comes on and says:

'Akownt numbuh?'

I'm not expecting this, so I ask her to repeat what she said.

'Your akownt numbuh. I need to know your akownt numbuh.'

In case you're trying to decipher what dialect I'm trying to convey, don't waste your time. I'm just expressing phonetically what I heard, as precisely as I can. I don't have a clue where it was from, but I guess we're talking London somewhere. We're sort of in Janet Street-Porter territory, wherever that is.

I find myself at these times very anxious to please because a chance remark, which I'd consider only mildly satirical but she might well regard as gratuitously offensive, can have me plunged to the back of the queue with the flick of a switch. With no redress. So I'm not going to say, 'Please don't bother to apologize for keeping me hanging on for half an hour listening to asinine music. I'm just a customer who pays the bills.' No, I'm going to try as hard as I can to stick to the rules.

'I'm sorry. I don't know my account number. I'm at work, but we have a power cut at our home in Kingston.'

'Woss the posscowd?'

I got it straight away this time and I spell it out. She doesn't understand me. I try again, and then again, and I briefly consider trying to render it in an impression of her accent, but feel this is too perilous. The back of the queue is just a click away. I try again, this time using some verbal aids, such as 'K for kilo, T for Tommy'. Eventually we get there and again I find myself having to resist the temptation to apologize for having to speak English.

'Behr wiv mee.' Click. Music.

Now I swear that this goes on for ten minutes. Not a word of a lie. Eventually I put the phone on speaker and treat the whole office to the aural torture. At one point the line crackled into life just long enough for the woman to say 'Behr wiv mee' again, but then clicked off before I got the chance to plead or remonstrate.

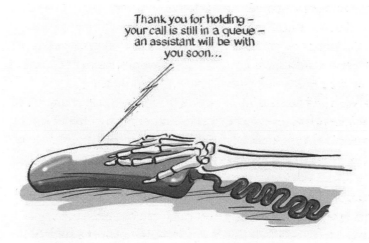

Thank you for holding –
your call is still in a queue –
an assistant will be with
you soon...

The agony comes to an end at last when she gets back on the line and says that, yes, there's a power cut. Someone has cut a cable in Turnip Road, or somewhere, and 88 houses are affected.

'Thanks; I already knew there was a power cut, but how long will it take to mend?'

She has no idea, but if I like someone will ring me when they have news.

I'm defeated.

I call my wife and I give her the bad news and ask her to call me if the power comes back on. Nothing happens for the rest of the afternoon, and six hours later I call my wife again to say I'm on my way home. She tells me there's no heating, the house is in total darkness, the contents of the fridge and freezer are probably all ruined and we've nothing to eat. Though to be fair, she does a pretty good job of not implying that it's all my fault.

As I'm getting nearer to home, I'm looking at the houses to see where the power cut starts, and am surprised to see lights on at the end of my road, in my road itself and, indeed, in every house except ours.

When I get off my bike my mobile phone is ringing and there is a message timed half an hour ago saying that the power should be back on. Oh Christ, I know what's happened and am having to think quickly about how to handle it.

The house is freezing. My wife is fed up. Being of an ultimately generous nature and romantically inclined, I say, 'Never mind, let's have a take-away by candlelight.' Then I go to the garage and flick the master-switch on the fusebox that has probably blown at the moment the power surged back on and thereby kept the house in darkness when everyone else had been reconnected.

'Why these companies don't simply employ enough people to answer the calls they get, I just don't know. I mean, there's nothing worse than picking up that phone, dialling the number and hearing that there's a queue now ... 35 minutes before they can answer your query. In many cases, I'm trying to give them money. Why should I wait 35 minutes to get someone who can explain to me how I give them money? Outrageous.'

JOHN STAPLETON

4 FEBRUARY

It's Lizzie's birthday later this month and she's told her mother that she'd like to have a party. She's told her mother, and her mother has told me. Lizzie hasn't told me herself, I gather, because she doesn't want me to have 'an epi'. That's the word she uses when I'm going off on one and she wants to irritate me even further. I'm not sure if it means 'episode' or 'epileptic fit', and I've never been calm enough when it's mentioned to enquire.

'That's great,' I say, 'where?'

'Here.'

'No way.'

'But she's about to be 16. Surely better for her to have these things here, where at least we can exercise some control, than to be out somewhere getting legless and doing drugs.'

I point out that we won't be able to exercise any control during the party because we certainly won't be allowed to stay in the house; and since they are all going to get legless and do drugs, I'd prefer this to happen somewhere else.

'This is the reason she won't talk to you about these things.' My wife wisely decides that it is better to let the idea sink in, and talk to me about it again later.

6 FEBRUARY

Was determined to go to Piss-Pots gym today for a swim. After all, it's costing me £10 a week and I haven't yet visited. I tried on my swimmers last night and was absolutely disgusted by the hideous image reflecting back from the mirror; nonetheless, they're the biggest pair I've got, so I wrapped them in my towel and took them with me to work. By this evening every fibre of my body wanted just to get home, stink the place out by grilling my Craster kippers, pop them on a plate with liberally buttered brown bread, and put my feet up in front of a recorded episode of *Six Feet Under*. But I thought, 'No, am I a man or a mouse?' So I made a 3-mile detour through the rush hour, got parked, queued to get in, only to be greeted at reception by a notice saying 'Pool closed for renovation'. My reaction was the perfect mix of outward fury and concealed relief. By heck those kippers were lovely.

7 FEBRUARY

How about this? Today I needed to drive to Kingston to get some keys cut, or something equally enthralling, when to my amazement both Matt and Lizzie said they'd like to come with me.

'What for?' I didn't mean it to come out sounding so suspicious, but it's so rare that either of them would do anything with me through choice that I had to wonder. But no, they both seemed genuinely a bit bored and wanted to come for the ride.

We parked up and both the kids walked with me as I went to find Mr Keyhole or whatever he's called on the corner of Market Square. I can't remember the last time this happened, and all was going fine until we passed HMV.

'Hang on, Dad,' said Matt, 'I want to go in here for a minute.'

I told him to catch up with me in the key shop, and kept going. I arrived at Mr Keystone, or whatever, who said he could cut the keys, but that he had a backlog and it would take two hours. Excellent. Not enough time for it to be worth going home and coming back, but more time than I wanted to spend in town; and also I'm going to have to go back and feed the meter.

So Matt is still in HMV and I'm at a loose end. Lizzie says we should have a walk round the shops. It's Saturday. I want to walk around the shops about as much as I want to join the Hitler Youth, but I'm aware that I don't spend enough time with Lizzie, so I say we'll go where she wants to.

First thing is that she wants to go into Big Face or Fat Arse or whatever it's called, but nothing is going to persuade me to go in there with a 15-year-old because I haven't showered or shaved this morning, and I'm fairly sure that everyone is going to look at me as though I'm a pervert. And who knows, I might discover that I am a bit of a pervert; which I don't want to do at all, and certainly not in front of my 15-year-old daughter.

So she doesn't want to go into the bookshop, and I don't want to go into the Stuff-Your-Own-Teddy-Bear Shop. Eventually it starts raining, she's getting a bit fed up, so I allow her to lure me into a gift shop.

Now these places are among my pet hates. You know exactly the sort of thing. Tiny, overdecorated shops crammed with pastel-coloured, joss-stick-scented, fabricated junk of every size and description in every nook and cranny, all to the musical accompaniment of dolphins farting somewhere in the far distance.

Recognize it?

If you are taller than the average hobbit, you're in constant danger of bumping into assorted wind-chimes or having an ever more elaborate 'dream-catcher' trailing across your head. 'Dream-catchers' – that's a good one, isn't it? When we were kids Red Indians whooped and hollered and lived in wigwams, but had the decency to keep on riding around the encircled wagons on their horses, firing futile arrows inside the circle while you picked them off with your Winchester. Occasionally, they cheated and evened up the score a bit by setting fire to the arrows, but usually we sorted them out in the end. You didn't hear much about 'dream-catchers' in those days. No sirree.

Anyway, now these items are among a million varieties of total crap, class C drug-related paraphernalia, shiny stones, fossilized sea creatures, little models of folk from the Shire and 'Aragorn, son of Arathorn, bearer of the sword', most of it smelling of incense or vanilla, and all of it overpriced. Stuff you'd be embarrassed even to put in your dustbin. It's an industry – a huge industry based on complete, total and unutterable bloody rubbish. And whale song.

So anyway, I'm in this shop, craning my head hither and yon to avoid cracking it on some low-flying Smaug, when Lizzie says: 'Do you think Mum would like one of these for Mother's Day?'

Now some days you might allow yourself to believe that you haven't done a bad job of bringing up your kids, and then something like this happens and all you can do is ask yourself 'Where did we go wrong?' I look around and she's holding up what looks like a bootlace with a shark's tooth attached.

The trouble is that I'm too close to the counter, and the new-age hippy with seersucker tie-dye and Ophelia haircut, to be able to say what I really think. Which is something along the lines of, 'Yeah, when there's been a nuclear holocaust and we're all back to the stone age and need something to cut the skin off a rabbit; that's when she might appreciate a shark's tooth pendant.' But instead I say, 'Maybe, but perhaps you should look around a bit more first.'

Anyway she bought it, then we got a text from Matt saying 'Where the fuck are you?' – nice to think we've brought him up so well – at least he added the question mark. We met him back at Mr Keystage, or whatever, got home and guess what – the keys don't work.

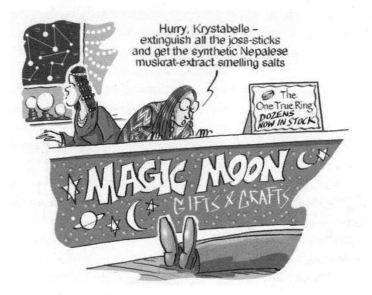

'Potpourri. I even find the name irritating. Potpourri. It must be great if you live in these villages – "Oh God, we're out of potpourri. Quick! Luckily we've got a shop that sells potpourri and vanilla-scented candles, so we're all right here." The other thing they sell, which is really useful, is little statuettes of Gandalf, or little painted Harry Potters, or little shaky snow scenes. And they say that Britain doesn't have a manufacturing industry any more. We don't build ships, we don't build cars, but we make these little Gandalfs and we lead the world in little shaky snow scenes of Big Ben. Actually no, they're made in China.'

JOHN O'FARRELL

11 FEBRUARY

It's very rare that a phone call at home is for me, and when it is it's usually bad stuff of one kind or another. About 50 per cent of the time it's news that a friend of mine – usually someone about my age – has died or has some terminal illness. That's happened today and the funeral is next week.

12 FEBRUARY

Robert Kilroy-Silk. All over the papers today because he's joined a party or left a party or attended a party or thrown a party, or something or other. Honestly. Where would you start? Be honest – have you ever come across more of a plonker in your whole life? What does he think he looks like?

Someone told me that he's handsome, and I guess I can see it – but honest to God, I'd rather be the bloke I am, with thinning hair, bloodhound eyes and drooping chins, than look like he does. I really would. But leaving aside his appearance, because maybe being orange is an affliction he can do nothing about, who on earth does he think he is? And why, oh why, does anyone on the television ever ask his opinion about anything? As if any of us could give a damn? I think I'd rather know what Cilla Black thinks about something than Robert Kilroy-Silk. So here's a piece of free advice to the people who run the TV news and current affairs. Robert Kilroy-Silk is of no interest to anyone. Stop following him around and stop interviewing him. Please.

14 FEBRUARY

I'll tell you what is sometimes a bit difficult if you're a bloke, and that's working out what the problem is. With your partner, I mean. Like on Valentine's Day. In a recent series we made for

BBC2 called *He Says, She Says*, Grumpy Old Man Tony Hawks talked about how he'd like to have a sort of invisible male jury alongside him to appeal to when he's offended his partner.

'So what did I do wrong?' They'd all scratch their heads, confirm that they might just as easily have said or done the same, and wouldn't have the slightest idea of the reason for the problem. The equivalent female jury, on the other hand, would say, 'Guilty as charged – 15 years'.

So here's one – buying flowers from a garage. When it's pointed out to me, I can sort of see why it's not a good idea to buy flowers for Valentine's Day from a garage or a supermarket, but I probably wouldn't have got it on my own. The male jury would acquit you straight away; the female jury would have you flogged.

So today I went out to buy red roses from the florist – at three times their usual price – and a couple of boxes of Guylian. Valentine's Day is one of the few festive occasions that I can be relied upon to get more or less right. Because it's uncomplicated. Flowers and chocolates. I like that in a problem.

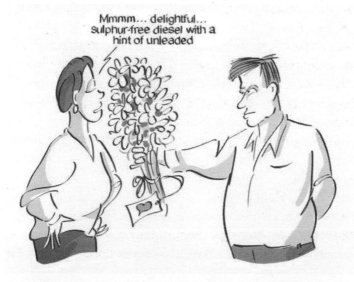

16 FEBRUARY

A story on the early evening news tonight about whatever is the latest political row between Labour and Tory. However, because this is about 'exchanging blows in the Commons' the reporter has come up with a wizard wheeze.

He's taken two boxers, dressed one in red and the other in blue, and they're sparring and occasionally landing blows on one another. Yep; we're in the ring with them, and we're being treated to a little staged dance by two obviously embarrassed blokes pretending to be sparring. Get it? Labour and the Tories exchanging blows.

Actually, the story also includes a role for the Liberal Democrats, but obviously they spoil the image, so they are represented by the referee – which doesn't really fit with what's going on. Inconsiderate of the Lib Dems, don't you think?

For heaven's sake, what on earth do these people take us for? Just tell us what the bloody news is.

17 FEBRUARY

We're always talking about how much communications and technology have changed in the 50 years or so that Grumpy Old Men have been on the planet, but I'm just as struck by how much rather more important things have changed – things such as funerals.

Today I went to the funeral of my mate who died last week, and I have to say that it wasn't much like the first funeral I went to in 1963 – for my grandmother. Her funeral involved a very substantial coffin made of mahogany, and a long row of hearses driving very slowly through the streets. At every junction the traffic stopped to let the procession pass, and on the pavement people would stand still and the men would remove their hats.

All the mourners wore black, many also with black armbands. All the women wore hats with black veils over their faces, and all wore gloves, as indeed they did for most occasions in those days.

The service went literally 'by the book', with no reference anywhere to my grandmother as an individual – and even at that young age I think I still remember a sense of relief from my mother that the vicar got her name right. We sang a few dirge-like hymns, the coffin was carried to the graveside and lowered in. There were plenty of tears, but they were subdued and dealt with discreetly.

We went back to our house. My mother served tea and my father served sherry. There were a few soggy sandwiches – probably tinned salmon because that was what constituted a posh sandwich in those days, hushed voices and then everyone went their separate ways.

Well, today's funeral wasn't much like that. No, not very much like that at all. It was early afternoon. Most people seemed to have come from work, and wore what they wore to work; in some cases, that included jeans and pullovers. There were no special cars, and the coffin – made of a material that looked like something left over from *Changing Rooms* – had already arrived, as if by magic. Since there are no hard and fast rules any more, no one really knew how to behave. Actually, they were all waiting for someone to 'break the ice' so that they could start laughing at an amusing thing the deceased person once said or did, and speculate on what he would have made of 'all this bollocks'.

The service consisted of a series of apparently off-the-cuff testimonials from friends and relatives, some of which were rather moving, but which sounded a bit as though they were more about the speaker than the deceased. Then there was a bloke with a guitar and his wife singing a strange sort of hip-hop version of 'My Way', which was alleged to be my mate's favourite song – though in 20 years I'd certainly never heard him say so. Outside in the car park everyone hugged and told jokes, and half went off to the pub to 'celebrate his life' while the other half went back to work.

On the plus side, no one sang a dirge, or mentioned an after-life (which I know he didn't believe in), and at least the service was in some way about him. On the minus side? Well, I don't know. Call me old-fashioned (and many people do), but I think I still want a bit of reverence when someone I know passes away.

Anyway, that's what's made me grumpy today.

18 FEBRUARY

Don't you just hate it when somewhere you've known all your life from geography lessons becomes somewhere else? News today that world leaders are meeting in Beijing. Not so long ago, that was Peking, and on the menu at the Chinese restaurant it still is Peking, but on the news it's Beijing.

But worse than that, much worse than that, was when Bombay became Mumbai. How did that happen? At least I can see a resemblance between Peking and Beijing. There's slightly less chance of being made to look an idiot by thinking they're different places. But how did Bombay become Mumbai? Or what about when Ceylon became Sri Lanka?

I know, I know, like everything else it's all our fault because in the colonial days we gave countries names that suited us. How arrogant can you be to name an entire country after some bloke you put in charge of it? Rhodesia. Eventually, when you kindly give the people their country back, they're allowed to call it what it should always have been. In cases like that I don't think I mind so much. Well, anyway, I know I'm not supposed to.

But then, doesn't it irritate you when people talk about taking their holidays in 'Murthia'? I always think they've got a lisp.

Then I realize they're talking about that place in Spain and have decided to pronounce it with what they think is a Spanish accent.

So when does this poncey rule apply, and when doesn't it? You don't hear people talking about going to 'Paree'. And when I was a kid, even posh people took their holidays in 'Madjorker'; so how come everyone and their auntie now goes to 'Mayorca'?

Yep, that's just another thing. Not a terrifically big thing, but still, it's another thing.

'I was watching the news the other day and they started talking about the "Gollam Heights" and I thought, hang on, is that in Toytown? I'd previously known them as the Golan Heights ... Yeah, they change the pronunciation now and again just to throw you off.'

ARTHUR SMITH

19 FEBRUARY

Oh, hell. A friend of my wife's has just returned from her holidays in the Maldives and reported it to be 'paradise'. Usually when this happens I point out some little-known drawback – such as that the government is unstable or they tend to have unexpected typhoons. The trouble in this case is that we've been to the Maldives before, and it is paradise. The only redeeming feature is that the sensible time to go to the Maldives is in the British winter, so I suggested that we keep it in mind in case we can't think of anywhere else we'd like to go. Close call.

20 FEBRUARY

I wonder which genius first thought it was a good idea to set the news to music. All that rippling, bubbling stuff that gurgles away under the headlines or summaries on BBC News 24 or whatever. At what moment did someone decide that '40 dead in Middle Eastern carnage' or 'Earthquake wipes out 1000 in Bangladesh' doesn't really sound sufficiently attention-grabbing? Let's add a bit of dramatic music so that people will know it's important.

And like everything of this kind, once one started doing it, they all started doing it, so that now the screen is cluttered up with countless countdowns and repeated resumés of what you've heard ten minutes earlier, complete with an under-current of drums beating momentously, cymbals crashing and every synthesizer sound effect with 'urgent' in its title.

This is necessary because we're all considered too stupid, with too short an attention span just to listen to a person telling us the news. And I guess we must be.

21 FEBRUARY

My wife raised again the question of Lizzie's party. Her birthday is on the 28th and it seems she needs a decision. I say that I've already made a decision – but it seems that it's the wrong one. I'm to be given a bit more time, apparently, to get used to the idea.

25 FEBRUARY

Well, I haven't made an entry for the best part of a week because, to tell you the truth, I've been laid up. That's what you call it when you get to our age. Laid up.

For the first few days I felt sure it was the flu. There's been lots of it about, and I had all the symptoms: head feeling like it's squashed under an anvil, limbs twice their normal weight but with no muscles to lift them, sweating like a Derby winner at night, all that charming stuff. Every day I felt sure I'd be fine and back at work tomorrow, and every morning I woke up feeling as though I'd been sleeping with my head under a walrus's arse, and took at least half the day to be able to sit up straight in bed.

So on the fourth day I started to do what we grumpies tend to do, and began to develop the conviction that I had something terrible. Meningitis … yes, I thought those lights were a bit bright. No sign of a rash, but now I come to think of it, it does feel a bit itchy over here. Or a case of bloaty head; now I come to really focus on it, I realize I can actually feel it growing under my cranium.

So I called the GP, who knows me well, and to his credit never lets slip even a hint of exasperation at my various eccentricities. He did all the usual tests, and I was just ready for him to tell me ever so patiently that I had a dose of the flu and would be better in a day or two when, instead, he said:

'I think we'd better get you to the hospital.'

This was a shock. I felt as though my bluff had been called.

'What've I got?'

'I don't know. Probably nothing, but just to be on the safe side.'

'What do you *think* I've got?'

'I don't know. I think it's best to let them have a look at you at the hospital.'

Now I hate this, don't you? You can tell he knows I've got something terminal, that I might not even make it to the hospital, but he doesn't want to say so. He's too nice a bloke. He doesn't want to be the one to break it to me. The first one to utter the dreaded words, 'I'm sorry to have to tell you this but … '

So now I wish I'd never called the doctor in the first place. This isn't what I had in mind at all. His job is to give a little reassurance, a little humouring, a little prescription, and to send me back to sleep. At home. Not to hospital.

So of course the thing you most want to do when you are feeling like shit is to get your clothes on, and go out in the driving rain and sit in the local hospital, but what choice do you have? Here's a bloke you trust saying you need to go. You can't really say, 'Oh, I don't think I feel so bad after all,' and anyway, I still felt at death's door.

So, being far too self-conscious to accept the offer of an ambulance, I insist that my wife drives me to the hospital, and here's the thing. When you get there, there's nowhere to park. Well, to be fair, there are a couple of public car parks, but you have to drive round and round for a long time to find a space, and then have a vicious stand-off with someone else who's been patrolling for as long as you. It's the usual battle of wills, except marked by the fact that you are both probably feeling sick, tired and desperate.

Once you find a space, of course you have to pay to park, and it's £1.80 per hour.

Now keep in mind that the government's target for waiting times in A&E is four hours. So in the unlikely event that you're going to be seen and dealt with within their target times, it's going to cost you £7.20 just to park the car. Which you have to do, not because you want to go shopping or walk by the river, but because you are ill. Too ill to get the bus, Ken, geddit?

So you pay for four hours' waiting time, and eventually get called in just as it's about to expire. You won't want to go and buy another ticket because you'll be missing at the crucial moment and lose your place in the queue, but if you go through the system, your time will have elapsed and you'll come out and face a parking fine – because you were late – because they kept you waiting longer than they were supposed to. Yes, this is the sort of crap that preoccupies grumpy old bastards all the time.

Even when you are turning up with an introduction from the doctor, as I was, and not unannounced off the street, once you find yourself checking in your details at A&E, you suddenly and totally change your status in the world. You are no longer a postman or an airline pilot or a salesman or a TV producer, you're a patient. Patients are there to go through the process. You have to go through the process.

But the problem is that it's an irredeemable feature of Grumpy Old Men that we don't like going through the process. Even when we are being put through the process by mostly very able, very committed, very well-intentioned people, we don't like it. And the worst thing is that you know yourself, that because you are a Grumpy Old Man, you are going to make things worse. For them. You're not intending to, you just are.

First of all you get to see the triage nurse, and of course she's really nice and really capable, and she's seen and heard in one shift more appalling behaviour and general bollocks than you'll probably ever see in your whole life. Nonetheless, she can't help herself. She talks to you about your symptoms as though you are a five-year-old and eventually says:

'Just wait outside. They'll call you for a fuller examination in a minute.'

I know it's a futile question but I can never stop myself.

'Any idea how long that will be?'

'It shouldn't be long. We're not very busy today.'

It's true that they aren't very busy today. There are a dozen people in the waiting room and none of them seems to have their head hanging off. So I go outside and wait. However, it becomes clear that her idea of 'not very long' is not the same as my idea of 'not very long'. My idea of 'not very long' is a maximum of about ten minutes. Hers has been refined and honed by years in the NHS.

I wait.

And wait.

And while you don't care, and why should you, all I can think of is that I have the headache from hell. All I want is to be in a darkened room with a towel wrapped tightly round my

skull and to be allowed to weep quietly into my pillow. Instead
I've got to sit on a hard metal bench, with the TV blaring, with
nothing to eat but junk food from a machine and nothing to
drink except from fizzy cans, for two and a half hours before
someone comes to call my name.

Then I go to a cubicle to wait some more.

So what happened was that over the space of the next four
hours, a succession of very able people said a variation of 'I'm
95 per cent certain that you have a virus, but just to be on the
safe side I want you to be seen by the doctor ... the registrar ... the
consultant ... ' At 6 o'clock in the evening, six hours after I arrived,
and now feeling a bit better, I'm still in the CDU – Clinical
Decisions Unit – waiting for the consultant to come round. And
there is no sign of him, and no one knows if or when he's coming.

So I say, ever so gently, to the very nice nurse: 'Look, I really
don't want to be a nuisance to anyone, but if it's OK, I think I'll
just pop off.'

'What do you mean?' I realize that she actually doesn't know
what I mean. Only people over the age of 45 ever 'pop' anywhere.

'I thought I might go home.'

She's genuinely confused, but I can see that this is a trigger
for a procedure she's been trained for. Part of 'the process'.

'Of course, if you want to go, we can't stop you, but you'd
have to understand that it was against medical advice, and we'd
need to get you to sign a form saying that you were leaving at
your own risk ... '

I want to just explain that I'm a Grumpy Old Man, and that
I just can't stay any longer. For us, being pissed about is like
Superman and red kryptonite; we've just got to get away. 'It's
just that there are a lot of very sick people here and I don't
think I'm one of them, so I don't want to waste your time and
my time.'

She's trying to be nice, and goes to talk to the ward sister.

I see a flurry of activity and faces turning in my direction, and this is what I've been dreading. I'm causing a fuss and I don't want to. I would have just slipped away, but would fear that this would precipitate a man-hunt and a knock at my door in the middle of the night from the bureaucracy police. Eventually the ward sister comes over and goes into a version of the same speech. I go into my version of the same speech.

Then comes the worst thing:

'If I get the consultant to come to see you now, will you stay to see him?'

'But then I'll be jumping my place in the queue and that's what I don't want to do.'

She doesn't have time for this. She goes off and brings him over. He is, of course, an urbane, totally delightful, conscientious man from somewhere exotic, and talks to me with total calm and total professionalism. Which makes me feel even more like a shit. He declares that he feels pretty sure that I'm suffering from a flu bug, but as I want to go home, he'll permit it (for which I'm pathetically grateful – as if I wasn't going anyway). However, he'd like me to come back next week for a little brain scan just to be on the safe side.

By this time I'll agree to anything – up to and including having a team of medical students peer up my arse with a periscope – just to get out of the place.

Seven and a half hours after I turned up (and £14 in the meter), I'm allowed back to where I really wanted to be the whole time. So there's no 'I'm sorry, I have bad news for you' this week, but maybe next. Who knows?

'On a Friday night it's like a field hospital in the Battle of the Somme. There's blokes with blood coming out of their heads and Bacardi Breezer bottles stuck in

their necks. It's just that A&E is now entirely devoted to looking after drunk people who've been fighting in the Red Lion car park on a Friday and Saturday night.'

JOHN O'FARRELL

26 FEBRUARY

Before all this I've never had any sympathy for people who stay off sick and say they have the flu. I always think of the flu as a heavy cold, and that if you were half a man, you'd get up and go to work. This experience has shown the error of my ways. Although I think I'm probably over the worst, I could no more get up and go to work than do the Great North Run on my hands.

However, I am feeling a bit better, so consequently am bored. Witless. Which has, of course, made me even more insufferable than usual.

I'm not ill very often, but I do feel sorry for anyone who has to be around me when I am. My pain threshold seems to be on a par with my boredom threshold. If I ever got anything really serious, I think I'd probably ask the whole family to go out for the evening and leave me with a large bottle of sleeping tablets. Save everyone all the bother.

Oh, and by the way, during my delirium I've apparently agreed to Lizzie's party on the 28th. Obviously, we're required to be out of the house. So that's just two days away. I feel like shit, and I have to find somewhere out of the house to amuse myself when all I'll want to do is bury my head in my pillow. Excellent.

27 FEBRUARY

Remember when films were films? Great epics, such as *Doctor Zhivago* or *Zulu*. Great romps like *Butch Cassidy and the Sundance Kid* or *The Sting*. Fabulous stories like *The Graduate* or *Papillon*.

What is it now? In her kind-hearted effort to alleviate my boredom, or perhaps more likely to shut me up for a while, my wife went down to Blockbusters to get some movies for me to watch. It's ages since we've hired anything so I felt confident there'd be a backlog of brilliant stuff.

She knows I usually like something with Al Pacino in it. Or Gene Hackman. Maybe Nicolas Cage or Andy Garcia. No point in getting anything with Clint in it because she knows I've seen them all hundreds of times.

Well, apparently they didn't have anything like that. For a start, everything seems to have Will Smith in it. Or if it doesn't have Will Smith, it has two cops, usually one white and one black, trying to out-mouth each other with smart-arse remarks. Or Jim Carrey; great facial expressions, but when you've seen one, you've seen them all.

There are also loads of disasters of one kind or another, which are basically just an excuse to show off a lot of visual effects. They're no doubt very clever, but again, when you've seen one tower block or dinosaur exploding, you've sort of seen them all. That's what movies are these days: no story, no script, hardly any acting – just a lot of slick smart-mouth kids with a repertoire of stupid faces and well-known buildings blowing up.

She comes back with something called *The Motorcycle Diaries*, which is one of those films you're supposed to think is good because it's got subtitles. Actually, it turns out to be pretentious shit. None of the people who went round saying they loved it actually did; it's the emperor's new clothes. I'd rather read a book. Which I do – which immediately sends me to sleep.

28 FEBRUARY

It's 6 p.m. and we're about to be packed off to spend the evening with Peter and Nicky because we're not allowed to be anywhere in the vicinity when Lizzie's friends arrive for her party. It's just like 40 years have rolled away and I can hear myself saying exactly the same words my father said to me. It was a waste of his breath then, and it's a waste of my breath now, but somehow you can't stop yourself, can you?

29 FEBRUARY

This morning the whole house looked like the scene of the Toxteth riots and smelt like the toilets at Glastonbury. Even though I wasn't at the party, I looked and felt as though I had been. I made an excuse and left early to go to work.

On my return home this evening, my wife met me at the door with a facial expression suggesting that there's been a death in the family. Cleaning up this morning, apparently, she found the remains of a joint under a chair. She thinks I should have a word with Lizzie.

'Saying what?' I'm thinking about our own youth, and just grateful that we haven't found lengths of rubber tubing and charred spoons.

'Well, obviously she's doing drugs. She's your daughter; I thought there was a remote possibility that you'd be concerned.'

I always know that action is required when my wife resorts to sarcasm, and I also note that Lizzie is always 'my daughter' when she's refusing to do her homework or staying out late, and my wife's when she's passing her exams. However, I'm guessing that this isn't the moment to point that out.

'OK, I'll deal with it,' I say, and all I'm thinking is that I won't.

March

1 MARCH

So today I had to go in to have my CT scan. Loads of 'jokes' at home about how they all knew I needed to have my head examined. It's always good to feel drowned in the milk of human kindness.

Mine was the first appointment of the day, at 8.45 a.m., so the great thing was that it couldn't be delayed. I turned up at 8.35 a.m. to be on the safe side, and the very nice woman said that the radiographer would be with me 'momentarily'. So I sat on a plastic stackable chair and flicked through the nine-month-old copies of *Reader's Digest* magazines. That took 15 minutes. Then I took a stroll around the notices on the board, which included a warning that I should tell the doctor if I might be pregnant, an appeal to donate my old specs and the confidential telephone number of the clinic for sexually transmitted diseases.

My mobile rang, and three seconds after I answered it the receptionist was all over me like a swarm of vampire bats warning me that it may well be interfering with the very equipment that I was about to use. The implication was that not only was I an inconsiderate bastard, but I was also putting myself and all those around me in danger. I rang off.

Twenty-five minutes after my appointment time, with only me and a Chinese woman in the waiting area, a strangely shaped radiographer emerged from a room and yelled my name at the top of her lungs. I looked over at the Chinese woman, determined that they couldn't mean her, and stepped forward.

Now of all the various things I suffer from, claustrophobia isn't necessarily one of them, but nonetheless, I wasn't really looking forward to having my head stuck in this tunnel. The strangely shaped radiographer said it would take five minutes and I should move around as little as possible, so I decided to see if I could concentrate on something that would divert me from my immediate circumstances. I've frequently thought that I don't really get quite enough quality time to devote to considering the various particular merits of the individual members of Destiny's Child, and so I thought this might be the opportunity for a catch-up. Anyway, to come to the point, I fell asleep.

The next thing I knew, the oddly shaped radiographer was congratulating me on remaining so still. She said she'd be sending the results to Dr Spleen, and that I should make an outpatient appointment to see him. As it happens, I know Dr Spleen; he's a gastroenterologist and he occasionally sticks his finger and other implements up my bum to make sure I'm not about to contract bowel cancer. See what I mean when I say I know him?

So anyway, I'm a big fan of Dr Spleen, but I couldn't work out why my brain scan would go to a gastroenterologist.

'Many people have told me over the years that I keep my brain up my arse,' I said quietly to the radiologist, 'and no doubt Dr Spleen would be amused to see an X-ray of my head for a change, but I can't help feeling that a mistake has been made somewhere.'

Somehow she managed to resist the temptation to fall about laughing at my hilarious joke, and instead consulted her file.

'Well, it was Dr Spleen who asked for the CT scan.'

'Sorry,' I said, 'but I'm afraid it wasn't. I know Dr Spleen; he treats me for other things. That may be why his name is on my file. The doctor who asked for the scan was Dr Watson. I know that because I was there when he asked for it.'

'Well, we have to send it to the doctor whose code is on the request form. That's Dr Spleen. It's a legal document. We can't do anything about it.'

I was perplexed. Plainly I was interfering with 'the process'. Being difficult. That's an unforgivable sin, for which the punishment is death by bureaucracy.

'Well, how about this? Could you send it to Dr Spleen, and maybe also send a copy to Dr Watson – on the off-chance that he's interested?' This was obviously a major departure from procedure and had the potential to totally fox the system. There was a lot of scratching of heads and murmuring in the corner. Eventually they said they thought they could do that.

'But it was Dr Spleen who asked for it.'

Whatever. I'll let you know what happens.

5 MARCH

Today my wife asked if I had had a word with Lizzie about the discarded joint we found after her party. Said I'd been waiting for the 'right moment'. She pointed out that the 'right moment' to ask your 16-year-old if she's been doing illegal drugs is the moment you suspect it. Reluctantly I concurred. Perhaps I will have to do it after all.

6 MARCH

It seems that those bastards whose job it is to ponce around the world having smoke blown up their arses by every major city stupid enough to want to host the Olympics are now in London.

By the time you read this, of course, the outcome of this particular piece of pestilence will be known and, like most right-thinking Londoners, I sure as hell hope it's going to Paris. Or New York. Or, indeed, anywhere but here.

I won't go into all the reasons, but for me the idea of all that bloody hoopla and bollocks is bad enough when it's clogging up someone else's doorstep. But having it near me would drive me crazy faster than I'm already going.

Anyway, the point today, apparently, is to demonstrate that London's transport system won't be a problem. Yes, that's right, you read it correctly. London's transport system won't be a problem. The system that collapses under the strain of a light flurry of snow or the wrong kind of fog will work fine as 40 million extra journeys (or whatever it is) are made in the space of a month.

So we've got reporters from the local news and reporters from the national news getting in their cars or on to buses and trains and testing different journey times to and from the proposed site. And yes, all of them are taking about the same amount of time as it would if they were walking. With a limp. Carrying a boulder.

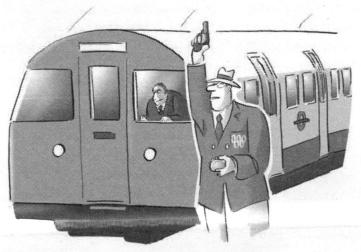

But here's what creases me about this. Who gives a shit about the massive everyday inconvenience, week in week out, month in month out, to all of us sitting there like sodding over-familiar sardines and smelling about as sweet? Who gives a shit? No one. But when it comes to the idea that sometime in the next decade a load of foreigners that none of us cares about might want to flit backwards and forwards to a stadium that will be used once, and then moth-balled for all time, we're all getting ourselves into a lather about it.

Have we gone mad or what?

7 MARCH

The subject of holidays came up again today. My wife said she'd been thinking about my suggestion of driving down the East Coast of the USA to Carolina, and thought she might like the idea.

'Maybe,' I said, as though I'd been thinking hard about it too. 'On the other hand, it's quite a long way, and therefore quite a long time in the car. I've been wondering if we shouldn't have a run around the West Country to see if we can find somewhere we'll eventually want to retire to.'

This is a bit below the belt because my wife is always mentioning that we should have started thinking about where we might want to retire to. I see her pondering it. We have achieved another postponement. Fifteen love.

9 MARCH

'Have you asked Lizzie about the dope yet?'

'Yes,' I said.

'And what did she say?'

'She said she didn't know anything about it. It couldn't have been any of her friends because none of them smokes dope.'

'And did you believe her?'

That's a hard one to answer because of course I haven't asked her, and she didn't say what I've just said she said.

'Yes, I think so. Probably we should trust her and leave it at that.'

Hmmm.

11 MARCH

Is there anybody on the planet, do you suppose, who can read the index of the *A–Z* unaided?

You have to wonder if these guys are having a laugh, don't you? I couldn't read the *A–Z* index before my eyesight started to go the way of all things. Now that I have to squint at the telly and put a pair of reading glasses on the end of my nose like a character out of Dickens when I want to read something, all I can make out is a row of blurs. A blurred row of blurs.

That would be bad enough, but, of course, half the time you're trying to read it in the dark. Because, being a bloke, you've refused the wife's entreaties to look at the map before you left because you feel you have a pretty good idea where it is. Halfway there you realize that something's gone awry, but you persevere. The traffic is bloody awful and you're stuck in a one-way system. You're crawling along, and somewhere deep inside you know you are crawling along in the opposite direction to the one you really need to be travelling in.

'She' wants to stop and ask someone, but you'd rather run out of petrol and have to walk to the service station than ask, and eventually you complain that they must have changed the one-way system, and you consult the map.

First of all, of course, you can't find it. I think I must own about 100 copies of the *A–Z*, but one way or another it's never where I need it to be. It's supposed to be in the glove compart-

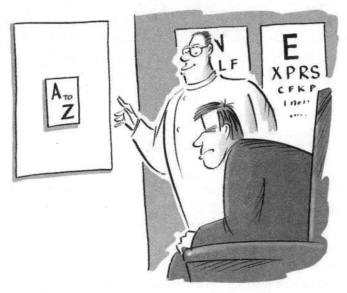

ment. No, that's full of the plastic cases of CDs you were given free with the Sunday newspapers, a can of de-icer, a scraper, half a packet of Trebor mints with fluff sticking to the one on the end, a small novelty torch, a dozen assorted yellow plastic bags that the parking tickets came in, and a broken pencil. Everything, in fact, except the bloody *A–Z*.

Is it under your coat on the back seat? You twist round to try to move whatever might be covering it up. Some cushion you put in the car six months ago for a long journey and that has been there ever since. No. Is it in the little pockets behind the front seats? You can squeeze your hand into the passenger side, but unless you're a contortionist there is no chance you can reach the pocket behind your own chair; but that doesn't stop you from practically dislocating your arm in the attempt.

Eventually, you find a copy stuffed halfway under the rubber floor mat and wipe off as much of the mud as you can before laying it on your lap. This one is in a ring binder and all the pages are crumpled. Eventually you find the index.

You move the bloody thing about, trying to get it into a shaft of light coming from somewhere, screw up your eyes, adjust your focal length by stretching your arm out in front of you until you hit the dashboard, and still you can't focus on the bloody thing. You put on the so-called 'courtesy light', which has the illuminating capacity of a candle in a hurricane, or try to catch a shaft of light from one of those yellow streetlamps.

No, there's nothing else for it; you're going to have to stop the car.

And search for your specs.

Even with my specs on, I'm honestly struggling to read the index. Squinting and contorting to try to decipher it. Eventually I do, and still can't find what I want.

Today (and this is why I'm writing this now), I wanted to go somewhere called Brook Place. Needless to say, I couldn't find it in the index, but that's because road names are in the wrong order. See if you agree; it goes from Brook Court to Brookdale Road and then Brook Drive. When I went to school you'd have gone from Brook Court to Brook Drive and only then on to Brookdale Drive – or is that just me?

Anyway, it turned out that Brook Place is off Lancashire Court, and not listed in the index. I arrived 20 minutes late, which I hate to do. All because of the sodding *A–Z*. So that's another thing.

'I've given up, I admit it, I've surrendered to it. I simply decide, well, where roughly do I have to be? And I go there and hope through some kind of osmosis I'm going to find where I'm supposed to be. It's no good giving me a map – it means nothing to me.'

DON WARRINGTON

12 MARCH

Needless to say, I've heard nothing yet about my brain scan. Mostly I want to believe that this is because it went straight to the right department, was examined by an international expert, who marvelled at the remarkable size, exquisite functionality and elegance of my brain, but could otherwise find no abnormalities. He therefore put it in the pile waiting for the 'everything's cool' letter to be written. That's what I want to believe.

What I actually believe is that the scan results went to Dr Spleen the gastroenterologist, who had no idea why he was receiving them and put them in his 'pending tray'; and they are also sitting in the pigeon-hole once allocated to Dr Watson, but who was only working as a locum that week and is now back in college in Barnet or something. Meanwhile, whatever the problem, it's growing at the back of my head.

But I don't believe this with enough conviction to brave an encounter with the hospital bureaucracy in trying to track the scan down, so I guess we'll wait a bit longer.

14 MARCH

An item on the 'news' today that London Underground is going to issue a badge saying 'Baby on board' so that pregnant women can wear it in the hope that people will give up their seats. It strikes me as an excellent idea. I'm going to have a badge made saying 'Six pints on board', and I guarantee that anyone who finds me standing over them will give up their seat like a shot.

15 MARCH

The early evening 'news' on ITN is getting more and more full of crap every day. They are reporting tonight that an elderly woman in north London seems to have been stabbed by a burglar. Is that how they tell it? Of course not.

It starts with the presenter looking at the camera with something he mistakes for a sincere expression on his face, and saying something like 'In an ever more violent world, some crimes still leave us floundering for an explanation.' Yes, yes, get on with it, what's the story? But there's more. 'From time to time we report on the ever-increasing violence in our everyday lives, but what happened today in an ordinary street just like the ones we all live in still leaves us in shock.' All right, we get the idea; now what the hell happened? But no, they're still not going to tell us.

We're then going over to the reporter at the scene, who has to tell us how this very ordinary street is in shock tonight with people asking how such a thing could take place in broad daylight. We zoom in to a shot of a tent in the front garden of what is, indeed, a very ordinary house in a very ordinary street. And they still haven't told us what happened.

How about this guys – you tell us the news, and we'll decide how shocked to be. Would that be OK? Probably not.

16 MARCH

Have you noticed that there are far too many people in the world, all getting in the sodding way? This week is half-term, and at such times you get an occasional glimpse of what the streets should be like. Such is the general level of prosperity these days that enormous numbers of people seem to jet off somewhere. We know this because every half-term, without fail, one group of arseholes or another at the airports threatens to go on strike. And when we hear about them on the news – the baggage-handlers, or the cabin crew, or the air traffic controllers – you always, without fail, hear people say, 'What bastards!

Fancy waiting till half-term when everyone wants to take their kids away for a holiday,' like that wasn't the point. Yes, folks, they're doing it deliberately at half-term because the general idea of the action is to piss off as many people as possible.

Anyway, one way or another, quite a lot of people these days find somewhere else to go during half-term rather than get in my way, and all of a sudden there are about 40 per cent fewer people trying to do the same things I want to do. I can more or less get to work. More or less park the car. More or less get in the cinema. More or less book a table in the places I want to eat.

Now this feels a bit more like it, I find myself thinking. If there were about half as many people in the world as there are, maybe life would be a lot less irritating. Then I start to ponder the various ways that this might be achieved, and even at my most misanthropic, most of them seem unacceptable. I therefore contemplate how I might find ways to disengage from this rat-race. After all, I'm 53 now. Having put up with it for what must be at least three-quarters of my life span, surely I must be due a break sometime soon? Do you think?

21 MARCH

Just got off the phone from what, for me, was an unusually long conversation with my mate Peter. To tell the truth, I don't have a lot of 'mates', and those I do have I don't spend a lot of time talking to on the phone. But he called up to tell me about an incident that perfectly illustrates the lot of the Grumpy Old Man.

Peter had to take his car into the garage for a service. He didn't have anything else particularly to do, but instead of taking his wife's advice and allowing her to pick him up and drop him off later, Peter had to have a courtesy car. After all, it was only £10, and it gave him a chance to have a fun drive around in a car he wouldn't usually have. So he chose a Jeep Cherokee.

So far so good.

No sooner does he leave the garage than he realizes that, of course, for a charge of £10 they won't have put any fuel in the tank, so he reckons he'll stop and put in just £10 worth because that's all he'll need.

He puts £10 worth of petrol in the tank, is just about to pay, when he realises that the Jeep is a diesel. Thank you, God. And if you're one of those people who is now thinking 'What a plonker. I would never be so stupid,' my view is that you are just asking for fate to bring down some shit on your head.

Anyhow, now as sick as a very bilious thing that's just eaten a Big Mac, Peter decides to call the garage on his mobile. Immediately the petrol station attendants come running out and start verbally beating him around the head and neck for causing a risk of an explosion. Apparently this has happened sometime and somewhere; someone making a phone call on a petrol station forecourt managed to blow up the whole bloody thing. So now Peter can't start the car and has to make his call from 50 yards away. And it's pissing down.

The garage tells him to call Jeep Recovery, but he doesn't want to do that because it'll take hours, and anyway he's only half a mile from them. Won't they come and tow him back so they can drain the tank? Apparently not.

Then Peter has an idea. He's only put £10 worth of petrol in an empty tank; maybe if he fills it up with diesel, the petrol will be sufficiently diluted that the car will run. If it works, it'll solve the problem; if it doesn't, it'll be five times the time and trouble to drain the tank. He takes the chance, putting in another £55 worth of diesel, making a total of £75 he's spent since he left home. He holds his breath. The engine starts. It runs fine.

Now Peter is pissed off. He's paid for all this fuel and doesn't really want to go anywhere. So his wife persuades him to drive into Salisbury, where he ends up buying a climbing rose and four pairs of gardening gloves that he didn't really want, for £70.

A day on which he could have spent nothing, but chose instead to spend £10, ended up costing £145.

I recount this because it represents exactly the sort of shit that comes along in our modern lives to make us more and more grumpy. Sure, it provides an entertaining anecdote for his mates, who will all be kind enough to take the piss out of him unmercifully for weeks to come, but for Peter it's just £145 pissed out of the window and yet another layer of liquidized cat crap overlaid on his daily struggle against the world.

23 MARCH

My wife told me today that Lizzie wants me to be a bit nicer to her boyfriend. Apparently, when he comes to the house he 'senses an atmosphere' and he suspects that I don't like him.

Of course I don't like him, but I'm genuinely confused about how he can have gained that impression.

'How can he have sensed an atmosphere?' I remonstrate. 'I haven't spoken more than ten words to him.'

'Could that be the point?'

Touché. 'But how can he sense anything? He wears a beany hat pulled down over his head, always has headphones in his ears, and comes through the front door and straight up the stairs without looking left or right.'

'That's because he thinks you're hostile.'

'I am fucking hostile. And why would he care anyway?' I remonstrate. 'Would you have cared at that age? Would I? Why does he want to get on with me? Does he want a round of golf? I don't think so. Or to go fishing? He's going out with Lizzie, not me.'

My wife tells me to calm down. Of course she's right, but really.

'Oh, and by the way, one other thing,' and I'm thinking

that this feels ominous. 'Your very frank and useful chat with Lizzie about the cannabis can't have had much effect because she says she can't remember having it.'

Ooops.

24 MARCH

Publication of the Rich List. How did that start? Does anyone in the world give a toss about the Rich List? Who's up, who's down? What could be more depressing? John O'Farrell thinks that the *Sunday Times* should publish the smug bastard list: 'We list the most conceited, self-satisfied, smug bastards, and at number one again it's Robert Kilroy-Silk. And they should do the other end of the scale,' he suggests. 'We publish Britain's top 100 people carrying a sign saying Massive Golf Sale.' Good idea John. I for one would find it more interesting.

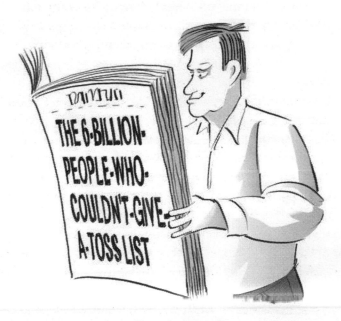

'Everything's a list now, isn't it? What was that programme I saw the other day – the 100 best celebrity mingers? I mean, that phrase alone strikes me as an analysis of what's wrong with Western civilization.'

ARTHUR SMITH

25 MARCH

Yesterday I decided that one of several reasons why I generally feel like shit for most of the day might be because I have an allergy to wheat.

Dunno what came over me – I must have been moping about the place and ended up reading one of those stupid articles by someone with sparkling eyes and shining teeth – you know, a sort of Rosemary Conley character – who was going on about allergies. Although I have no allergies that are immediately identifiable as clinical, I am allergic to so many things in every-day life – you know, David Owen, dogs, men with multiple piercings, etc. – that I figure I'm likely to be someone who has a few dietary ones.

Anyway, whoever it was writing this article was going on about the symptoms of an allergy to wheat, and they included tiredness, insomnia, listlessness, irritability, flatulence ... all of which characterize me perfectly. So I thought, maybe that's me. I could give up wheat, lose weight, sleep better and go around like one of those fit, shiny people I see on the telly or in magazines.

So that's fine. No bread then. No toast. No cakes. No Puffed Wheat or Golden Grahams. All very good, but what do you have for your breakfast?

Yesterday I looked in the fridge for a very long time, saw nothing that inspired me, walked around the kitchen, read the paper for a few minutes, and then went back to have another look in the fridge. As though someone might have been shopping in the interim.

Surprisingly, there was nothing new in the fridge since I last looked, so I ended up having a boiled egg. But a boiled egg is a bit much without toasted soldiers.

This morning I had porridge (or 'porage', as I am amazed to see it spelt on the side of the packet), but that felt far too healthy, so mid-morning I had a Twix and consequently felt like do-dos. Breakfast is a bit of a problem.

Much worse, though, if you're trying to avoid wheat, what can you do for lunch? Even when I'm not trying to avoid wheat, I get bored going into one of the thousands of sandwich shops that crowd out every high street. And the reason I'm bored is because there are far too many decisions to make.

The people serving in these places are always rushing around like lunatics, and seem to be either asylum seekers or foreign students. And because they're running around like mad things, you feel under pressure to have your order right on the tip of your tongue when they get around to asking you what you want.

Such is my general sense of ennui, that when this happens I sometimes ask them what they've got, or, even more provocatively, what they recommend. They look at me with the same sort of expression that Will Smith used a lot when encountering the aliens in the movie *Men in Black*, and once they've worked out that my response isn't consistent with any of the 50 words of English they've learnt – i.e. it doesn't include the words 'cheese' or 'ham' or 'chicken' or 'tuna' – they usually jerk their heads towards two huge blackboards attached to the wall above the counters, and get on with serving the next alien.

You look up and try to make head or tail of the scribblings. 1) is cheese, ham, lettuce, tomato and coleslaw; 2) is cheese, ham, lettuce, tomato and mayonnaise; 3) is cheese, ham, lettuce and tomato without coleslaw or mayonnaise. In short, there are hundreds of choices, mostly distinguished from each other by only minor adjustments.

So you choose one. Prawn, avocado, lettuce and tomato. Then, if all that effort hasn't made you lose your appetite, you have to choose the bread. Typically, you have a choice of white, brown, wholemeal, bap, French loaf or ciabatta. So bereft of stimulation is my life that once, when sitting on a bar-stool eating my sandwich recently, I worked out that if you took all the possible ingredients and all the available types of bread, there were 6.5 million alternative sandwiches in that shop – 6.5 million alternatives – and that's just lunch. In one shop. No wonder we're all overtired.

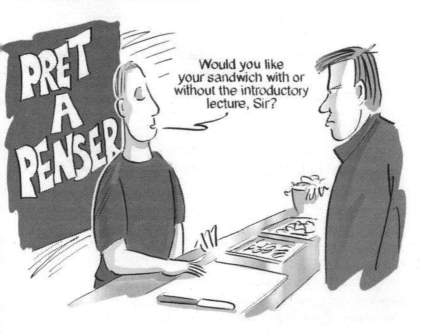

26 MARCH

The bank statement came in today and my wife asked, 'What's this standing order to Piss-Pots Gymnasium?'

'It's my gym membership. Remember I said at Christmas that I thought I should start going?'

'But you haven't started going. What you've done is to start paying.'

'I know, I know, I tried to go but the pool was closed.'

'Yes, but it's now the end of March and you've been paying for three months and haven't been once.'

I know she's right, but I hate having things pointed out to me that I know only too well myself, so I try to turn it back on her. 'I thought you'd want to encourage me.'

She looks skywards. Like the Piss-Pots Gymnasium who took my money knowing that I'd never turn up, she knows me too well.

27 MARCH

You'd think, wouldn't you, that if you were reliant on the good-will of others for your next meal, you'd try very hard not to get up their noses. So how is it that anyone who wants you to give them money can be stupid enough to sit on the pavement next to the cash machine? Do you know anyone that isn't driven to distraction by this practice?

You're queuing up in the pouring rain, hoping against hope that the cash machine won't have jammed or run out of money when your turn comes, and right alongside the machine is a bloke sitting on the pavement.

I don't really have a policy on beggars – sometimes I give them money and sometimes I don't. But what I'd never do is to give money to someone who's obviously trying to make me feel embarrassed about the fact that I can take cash out of a hole in the wall and he can't.

Almost all of us think it, but very few of us actually say it. However, the legendary Janet Street-Porter told us in *Grumpy Old Women* how she berated one such bloke along the lines of:

'Everyone in this queue has worked for the fucking money they're taking out of this machine, so why should they give it to you when all you are is an idle slob who should go and get a job and earn your own money.'

Way to go, Janet.

29 MARCH

Listened to a discussion on the radio this morning in which a whole load of air-head politicians were talking about 'choice'. 'What people in this country want,' said the Labour person whose name escapes me, and as though he had the slightest idea what people want, 'what people in this country want is choice.' Like it's an end in itself. 'They want to choose the best schools for their children. They want to choose which hospital they want to have their operation in.'

Then the equally forgettable Tory said more or less the same thing. Then the Lib Dem said something so flaccid that I went to take a leak.

And while I was standing there waiting to take a piss (I never used to have to wait to take a piss, but one of the many joys of late middle age is having to do so), I thought, 'What a load of old bollocks'. As you do.

People in this country don't want a choice of schools for their kids. How could that work anyway? You live in a small town, there are two schools, one of them is better than the other, and you want your kids to go to the better one. But not all the kids in the town can go to the best one. So they have to go to the other one, except now they're pissed off about it. What sort of choice is that?

Or you live in a suburb. There are two hospitals within a radius of 10 miles. One has a far better reputation than the other, but not everyone can get in there. What exactly is the choice you're making?

No (and by this time, you'll be relieved to know, I was urinating – slowly, but with purpose), what politicians need to get into their thick, stupid heads is that people in this country don't want a choice of schools or hospitals. *They just want the school or hospital near their house to be decent.*

Recently I read in the paper that the NHS was celebrating because it was close to its goal of achieving an average of not more than a four-hour wait in A&E. Yes, that's what they said. An average of a four-hour wait in A&E – and they want us to be grateful.

So you go in at 8 o'clock in the morning, with your ruptured appendix or split head or kidney stone, and if you're lucky, you'll sit there in agony or with blood gushing out of your fore-head for just 240 minutes before you get seen. I don't think, by the way, that four hours is the time you'll wait until you receive proper treatment; it seems to be the time you'll wait before you are bundled on to a stretcher and left in a corridor for 36 hours while people with clipboards pretending to be extras from *Holby City* run past. Four hours. It's a *target.*

Now once again, I think there is a basic misunderstanding here between the politicians and the people. If the former think that being close to achieving an average waiting time of four hours in A&E is a cause for celebration, I think they've got a problem. I don't think that's what ordinary people think is a cause for celebration at all. I think that's the average length of time they'd expect to spend waiting in A&E if they fell ill in Kabul. Not if they fell ill in what we are constantly being told is the fourth biggest economy in the world.

Let's do it in 'read my lips' language so that any politicians can understand it. People in this country want to: a) be allowed to kill anyone who burgles their house; b) get to work without enduring 1000 obstacles in the road, traffic jams, parking problems, overcrowded buses, trains and tubes; c) send their kids to a decent school close by; d) if they get ill, be treated in a local hospital with decent and friendly staff, and stand a reasonable chance of recovering and emerging fit and well, without succumbing to a superbug; e) be able to walk the streets without being vomited on by louts. Not necessarily in that order.

So how hard can all that be? Five things; well, six if you include never having to listen to Michael Howard talking on any subject, which would be a personal favourite of mine. Six simple things. But we sit there, listening to these jumped-up tossers talking bollocks about 'choice' or whatever is their latest drivel year after year after year, and then, when the election comes around, we're supposed to go out and vote for them.

31 MARCH

Since my conversation with the wife last week, my membership of the Piss-Pots Gym is weighing heavily on me. It's the end of March, I've so far paid them well over a hundred and fifty quid, and in my heart I know that I'm never going to go. So today I had what I thought was the bright idea that I might transfer the membership to Matt or Lizzie.

I haven't quite forgiven Lizzie yet for grassing me up (geddit?) to her mother over the joint, so I thought I'd start with Matt. Recent conversations with him have been confined on his side to a glottal stop or an occasional polysyllable such as 'Goin' out', but I was genuinely optimistic that this suggestion might lead to some dialogue.

'Would you like to take over my membership of the Piss-Pots Gymnasium?' I ask him.

'Do what?' is his charming reply.

'My membership of the gym. Do you want me to transfer it into your name?'

'You're a member of the fucking gym?' He is incredulous. 'Since when?'

Well, at least he can speak a sentence, I console myself, trying to resist the temptation to ask him not to swear in the house.

'Since January.'

Now he's still incredulous but also highly amused.

'You? The gym?' He walks off, shaking his head and laughing quietly to himself. So not such a great idea, then.

April

1 APRIL

So, how are we doing? We're about three months into this year which is supposed, if the Grumpy Old Men theory is correct, to see me starting to mellow. According to statistics, 35- to 54-year-old men are the grumpiest of any in history, and I'm coming up to 54 at the end of the year. After that, we're supposed to start taking it a bit easier. Becoming more accepting and acquiescent. Rolling with the punches. Going with the flow and all that bollocks.

And even leaving aside the hope that getting a bit older in itself might make me start to become a bit more mellow, there was always the hope that 'getting it all off my chest' might. How many times have we men been asked why we won't just talk about it? 'Get it out in the open. You'll feel *soooo* much better.'

Our answer to that is that we don't really want to talk about it. We want to bottle it up in our own fevered heads and deal with it. Like men used to do. Did Alan Ladd have to 'talk about it'? Richard Widmark? We don't think so.

Against my own best instincts, and anyway for the sake of the TV series, I did talk about it. Indeed, it seems I've done nothing but talk and write about all the stuff that gets on my tits for the last three years.

Has it been cathartic? Has 'talking about it' made any of it any better? Made any of it go away? Made any of it less of a pain in the gulliver?

Of course it hasn't. If anything, it's made it worse. Before I used to talk about it I was blissfully unconscious of the extent to which the stuff that is there just to irritate us joins up to form a continuous theme underlying our existence. How one irritation leads almost seamlessly to another so that grumpiness ends up being the perpetual state of our world.

No, talking about it has made it worse, and there is no sign whatever of creeping old age calming me down. Not yet anyway.

'There are days when it hardly takes more than a trip to the shop to buy the newspaper and in your mind you're saying, "Oh, look at this bloody traffic" or "Why don't they put a bollard there" or "God, how long do these lights take to change" or "Look at him in his stupid great big tank of a car driving along Barnes High Street – he doesn't need that". This is just crossing the road.'

ARTHUR SMITH

4 APRIL

Choice. Yes, yes, it's a week later and I'm still in a state about idiotic politicians talking about choice; and that's because this morning I tried to call an old mate of mine who left a message on the answering machine telling us he'd moved and asking us to call back, but was too terminally stupid to tell us his new phone number. And, before you ask, the 1471 facility said 'number withheld', which I always assume means that the person calling you also spends a lot of time making obscene phone calls.

Do you remember when you contacted directory enquiries by dialling DIR? No? Not old enough? Well, at least you must remember dialling 192. You wanted a phone number, you dialled 192, a rather short-tempered person on the other end asked you the name of the person you wanted, their initial, where they lived, and then read out their number to you. You'd write it down on a piece of paper, dial the number and speak to the person you'd enquired about. Quaint, huh?

Then someone decided that what we needed was choice. Competition. It's good for everyone apparently. So they closed down 192 and opened up a free-for-all. All of a sudden there were hundreds of variations on a 118 theme. David Bedford lookalikes running around – until David Bedford sued and the ads had be pulled. You remember. Idiotic jingles going round your head. 118 118. 118 500, 118 888 or whatever.

Does anyone know how many of these services there are now? Believe it or not, there are more than 500. That's right, we've gone from one to 500 with nothing in between.

So now we've got choice and guess what? Someone in Calcutta answers your call by asking you 'Which town?' You're not really ready for that, so you say, 'I beg your pardon?' 'Which town?' 'I don't really know which town – it's somewhere near Dartford in Kent.' They don't know Dartford from Rawalpindi, so they say, 'What name?' 'I beg your pardon?' 'What name?'

Eventually you narrow it down to an approximation of the person you're after and they ask, 'Do you want me to connect you?' And if you say yes, they say, 'That'll be 60p per minute' and then click off the line instantly before you can say, 'Are you fucking mad? Sixty pence a minute extra on my already extortionate call charges just because you've flicked a switch? Get real.'

Or if your wits are sharp enough to say 'No thanks', you go on to a recorded message that reads out the number, and even as

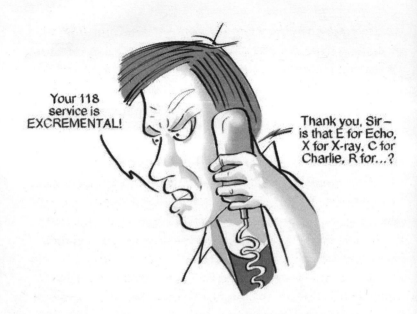

you are trying to write it down with the phone in one hand and the paper moving about under your pen, you have a feeling this isn't the right number. And guess what, it isn't. Last time I looked these services were giving out the wrong number one time in five, and 70 per cent of calls to directory enquiries cost more than the old 192 service.

So then you have to dial again. Is there any point in saying that you gave me the wrong number last time, so I don't want to be charged for that call? Of course not. You just go through the rigmarole again, and again, until eventually you give up.

That's choice for you. That's competition. Bring back 192, I say.

'I did get through once and they asked me, "Would you like us to put you through?" And I thought, "Well, I've just rung you for the number", presumably it's because I

want to ring it." It made me feel very old ... like a doddering old man. "Would you like me to help you cross the road?", "Shall I put you through?" And I say, "No, no thank you, I can do that.'"

DON WARRINGTON

5 APRIL

Came downstairs this morning to find the kitchen floor covered in enough feathers to stuff a double mattress. Yes, it's spring, and some poor family of birds, just trying to get started on the housing ladder and get going with the brood, have had their equivalent of a visit by the Yorkshire Ripper.

Naturally, I find this an excellent start to the day. There's nothing like clearing up bits and pieces of disembowelled bird first thing of a morning.

6 APRIL

And if that wasn't enough, in the early hours of *this* morning, suffering from my usual bout of insomnia, I eventually got so hot and restless and thirsty and pissed off with myself that I decided to go downstairs for some water. My wife is a light sleeper and even the flick of the light switch can be enough to wake her, so I tiptoed down the stairs in the dark. The very amusing Darth Vader slippers Lizzie bought me for Christmas have the obvious disadvantage of not being luminous, so I ended up going down in my bare feet. Walking across the kitchen, I suddenly found my left foot sliding away from beneath me, and was on my way to a heavy bodily crack on the tiled floor when my elbow collided with the worksurface and broke my fall, but very nearly broke my bloody arm as well. Cursing loudly, I scrambled to the light switch to find that I had slipped on the regurgitated remains of said bird or birds from yesterday's meaningless slaughter. Yesterday the raw stuff, today the same basic material but half-digested and smeared across the bottom of my left foot. Oh, the unequalled joy of keeping cats.

And yes, it woke my wife up.

7 APRIL

For the last week my wife has been urging me not to buy her any chocolate for Easter. If I were to heed this suggestion, it would indeed be a first. She is an addict, pure and simple. Chocolate to her is like cocaine, and the only way she can stop eating it is not to have it in the house.

Ordinarily, I would take no notice of this and would go ahead anyway and buy an egg or two. After all, it's Easter and, as Will Self so vividly put it in our *Grumpy Old Men at Christmas* special, the Lord Jesus so loved chocolate.

However, this time she really sounds as though she means it. She really does. She's saying things like, 'I know I always say this, but this time I really mean it.' Which could be taken to mean that she means it. Even more convincingly, today she suggested that I should buy her an orchid instead. 'I really do mean it this time,' she repeated.

Who knows, maybe she does.

8 APRIL

There are two things that get up my snitch about Easter. The first is Easter eggs, and the second is caravans.

Let's start with eggs, shall we?

Now last time I looked, Easter was about the Crucifixion and Resurrection of Jesus Christ. All that epic movie stuff about hauling the cross up the hill, barbaric death, Roman soldier having second thoughts, horrible weekend for all concerned, and then that 'rolling away the stone' saga. Great story. Most important weekend in the Christian calendar.

So how could we properly celebrate such an event? Well, obviously we could go to church, but that seems a bit dull, and anyway isn't much of a marketing opportunity. Hot cross buns? Yes, that's a good one. We've thought of those. Toasted and with plenty of unsalted Lurpak on mine, please.

No, the obvious thing to do is to celebrate Christ's death and resurrection with chocolate eggs. Big ones and small ones. Solid ones and hollow ones. Milk and plain, mint and creme-filled. Millions and millions and millions and millions of them. And the alleged rationale? Because an egg is a symbol of new life.

Bollocks. The reason is that once Christmas and the opportunity to sell crappy selection boxes is over, the chocolate manufacturers need a 'next thing'. Mother's Day isn't a bad one, but Easter is the real opportunity. And it can't come soon enough. Easter eggs appear in the shops in January and fill up more and more shelf space until a week after Easter, when you can buy them at a 50 per cent discount.

So why would I care? Well, I don't really, except that it's another 'thing'. Because what you pay for is all that crappy novelty packaging, while the chocolate in Easter eggs is, almost without exception, shit. It tastes like the stuff they scraped off the bottom of the vat after the real chocolate has been brewed. Horrible texture, vile aftertaste, not really justifying the name 'chocolate' at all.

So if it's not bad enough to have turned a solemn religious occasion into a cynical marketing opportunity, they're also doing it with a product that looks and tastes like the devil's shite. They're all going to hell, mark my words.

And the other thing about Easter is caravans. I wonder what it is about caravans that brings out the worst in everyone who doesn't own one? So many things, but uppermost among them the fact that, at the front of every traffic jam, there is some git who's taking his caravan out for its first stroll of the year. A bloody huge, white plastic thing on wheels, usually being pulled by a 15-year-old car that is obviously nowhere near powerful enough to cope with it. An Austin Princess or some sort of Maestro. The result of which is that they're going along at about 20 miles per hour, and taking up a lane and a half so that no one can overtake.

Yes, Easter eggs and caravans; both making their contribution to wrecking what might otherwise be a perfectly good bank holiday.

11 APRIL – EASTER SUNDAY

Well, guess what? She didn't mean it after all.

This morning my wife stayed in bed till 9 a.m., as is her habit on Sundays. This just gives me about five hours to kill before I can rattle around the house without care or discretion, and I usually use half an hour of it to go and get the papers. Today I made some breakfast at about 9.30 a.m. and took it in to her on a tray. Tea, toast, the newspaper and, yes, an orchid.

To be fair, she seemed genuinely delighted by the orchid, and I was delighted that she was delighted. She put it on the table so it could catch the light; then she admired it from a couple of different angles.

See if you can guess what happened next.

'OK, you've had your fun; where is it?'

'Where's what?'

'Don't mess about. Easter Sunday. What have you done with it?'

By now I'm getting alarmed. I've read about the dangers of an addict who's expecting a fix that isn't coming.

'I hope you don't mean "Where's my egg?"'

'Stop messing about,' she says, 'I know you've got me one.'

Well, I'll leave the rest to you. Fifteen minutes later I was back with the only Easter egg left in the local shop – a crappy Black Magic one that no one else apparently wanted.

You'd think I'd know by now, wouldn't you?

15 APRIL

I reckon that as a nation we're divided about 50/50.

Just about half of us are doing our very best to go about our everyday lives – fighting to get to and from work every day, sweating our bollocks off to earn enough money to try to keep our families off the streets, and body and soul together, keeping at bay the banks, the creditors, paying the mortgage, the payments on the car, the rates, the VAT and the congestion charge.

And the other half is trying to fuck us over.

Don't you find that? It seems to me that everything I want to do, some bastard somewhere is trying to make it harder for me. And apparently taking pleasure in it.

Just think about how all this started. Early society. Good heavens, we all seem to want to live close to one another, we'd better have a few rules. OK, we can't kill one another, and can't half-inch each other's stuff. All right? Everyone agreed? OK good.

That works for a while, but then it seems that there's a lot of coveting of thy neighbour's ox or whatever going on, so everyone agrees it should get a bit more complicated. 'Oi you, no coveting.'

'I wasn't coveting.'

'You were, I'm going to fetch a policeman.'

'Yeah? Well, policemen haven't been invented yet, so to hell with you.'

Oh yes, that's right. Policemen haven't been invented yet.

It's all getting a bit more complicated; better get a few people whose job it is to enforce the rules.

Then a bit later it's all getting more complicated still and we need a few more rules.

'Well, I haven't got time to be making a lot of rules. Tell you what, you make the rules and we'll stick by them.'

'What? I'm going to get to make the rules and you're going to do what I say?'

'Yes, that's right. We're too busy. So long as you don't start making any stupid ones, like forcing us to wear seat-belts in the back of cars.'

'No, no, of course we wouldn't be stupid enough to do anything like that.'

So that's how it started. Next time you look, there's hundreds of them. Thousands. All making up and enforcing rules for the rest of us, and we're too busy getting on with stuff to say 'Hey, wait a minute … '

Take something as simple as trying to go to work by car.

Let's leave aside for a moment all the bollocks involved in buying the car, registering it, the road tax, insurance, the petrol, the MOT, being messed about by mechanics … Let's leave all that to one side.

Before you get to the end of your street, someone has put a sleeping policeman in the road to give you the choice of slowing down or ripping the bottom out of your car, or has erected an obelisk sticking halfway out into the road, forcing you to swerve into the path of an oncoming vehicle.

When you reach the junction no one will let you out into the traffic, and when you eventually tire of waiting and take your life in your hands, an obese arse-head with a tight collar and high blood pressure in a BMW will blast his horn at you, flash his lights and maybe yell 'Wanker' out of the window – his hand gesture suggesting that his penis is far bigger than is plausible given the car he's driving. You'll shout back, 'What am I supposed to do, wait till hell freezes over?', give him the finger and then lock the doors, hoping that he won't still be behind you at the next traffic lights.

You'll proceed at the pace of a salted slug towards your destination, choosing every 20 yards whether to allow a 4 x 4 with Chloe and Tarquin on board out of the junction. When you do stop and wave someone out, they swing out in front of you without acknowledging your act of unnatural generosity, thereby making you far less inclined to assist the next poor sod trying to get out in front of you.

Somewhere en route you pause long enough at the traffic lights to send the text paying the congestion charge, and a policeman pulls alongside you and gives you a load of abuse for not paying attention to the road.

When you eventually get to the office, there is nowhere to park. You go round and round and round the streets, passing hundreds of empty spaces marked 'residents parking only'. Eventually you find a meter and park the car. The rate on the meter is 20p for five minutes. Yes, yes, I know, if you live outside London you don't believe it, but I swear it's true. Even to be able to carry enough change to feed the meter would involve giving yourself a hernia or using a wheelbarrow. You have to put about £17 into the meter for an average working day – or would if you were allowed to park in the same place for more than two hours.

As it is, you're going to have to return to the car every two hours and move it. Sometimes you'll be able to move it a few yards to the next bay; more often than not you'll have to drive round and round and round the block until you find another meter. And then start feeding it …

If you get back to the car one minute after the time bought, or if your wheel is 2 inches over the white line, you'll find a

fixed penalty notice charging you £50 if you pay within a fortnight, and £100 if you don't.

This is all so you can get to work to earn the money to pay
the tax to pay for all the obstructions we've just described. And
the shit-heads who dream them up.

Anyway, the point is that there is a whole industry – nay, a
whole series of industries – staffed with people whose job it is to
thwart the rest of us. And about half the people of Britain work
in them.

Think about it. There are all the people in the Inland Revenue
plotting and scheming to take your hard-earned money from you.
All the people administering the National Insurance, which was
originally supposed to insure you against unemployment or ill-
health and is now just tax. All the people in the VAT office taxing
anything you want to buy. All the customs people stopping you
from bringing in a little something you picked up for personal
use in an Amsterdam café (no, I don't mean Gerda, I mean a little
Lebanese blue, or whatever you call it). There's all the people in
the town hall stopping you changing the windows of your house
or building an extension on the back or parking within a half a
mile of your home. Or maybe they've decided it would be fun
to delay the traffic for three months on a main arterial route
because someone thinks it would be nice to rebuild the traffic
island. Then there are all the traffic wardens stopping you
parking where you want to. The police moving you on if you
pause to pick up the missus. All the guys from the gas board, the
electricity board, the water board, BT and the cable telly people
digging up the road. And that's before we get to the politicians …

So I've come to the conclusion that this is a good part of the
reason why the half of us who aren't thus employed, are
grumpy. We're just trying to get on with our lives, and we're
being thwarted at every turn. By the other half.

Think about it.

'I think it's quite possible that there's a government department somewhere devoted to coming up with really annoying ideas. You know, let's not have fresh pints of milk on trains any more, let's have those little cartons of UHT because that'll piss everybody off. Let's have car keys made bigger because those little ones fitted so easily into people's pockets. Let's make sure that maps don't fold up properly.'

JOHN O'FARRELL

19 APRIL

Woke up at 3 a.m. wondering why pants come in pairs but a bra is a single item. That doesn't make sense, now does it? And if pants come in pairs, what would one single pant be like? A last gasp? See what I mean? I'm far closer to insanity than may be obvious.

20 APRIL

Dunno if you've been watching GMTV lately – and I'm aware that these guys come in for an unfair amount of stick – but I ask you.

Recently they've been giving away cars, holidays with spending money thrown in, £10,000 in cash, or even villas in Spain.

What they do is run a nice little film in which a C-list celebrity shows us how jolly it is in Andalucia or wherever, and then you have to answer a question to enter the competition.

Now you need to understand that the rules laid down by the TV regulators insist that there must be an element of skill to

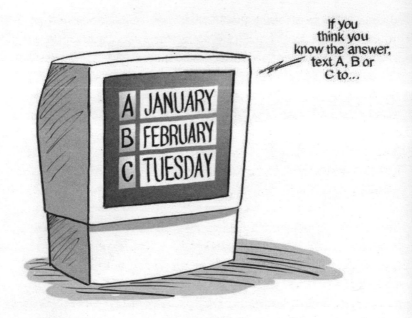

these questions – so the TV company can't just ask you what your name is. On the other hand, because you have to pay to enter, they want to encourage as many people as possible. So typically they'll ask something like: 'What is the capital of France? Is it a) Moscow, b) London or c) Paris?'

Then, and this is the killer, they say, 'If you think you know the answer, you can phone or send a text to us on … '

This is great, isn't it? 'If you think you know the answer.' Wherever possible, they'll make it seasonal. Over Christmas, for example, we had some festive alternatives. 'What colour Christmas was Bing Crosby dreaming of? Was it a) brown, b) green or c) white? If you think you know the answer, you can phone or send a text to … '

When I see this, I can't help but envisage the scene in the house where indeed they think they *do* know the answer to the Bing Crosby question. And presumably they believe they've already improved their chances of winning by a factor of three because so many other people will think Bing sang about a brown or a green Christmas. Already they're practically sunning themselves on the veranda of the new villa in Spain.

So they text in the answer. That costs £1 plus whatever are your operator's call charges. Or they phone – no doubt costing about the same, but with that option you get the thrill of listening to a patronizing voice talk to you as though you are a halfwit for a couple of minutes. Which of course you are, or you wouldn't have phoned.

So let's imagine – I don't have the real figures – but let's imagine that 10,000 people do this every day. Obviously, the commercial sponsor of the competition is providing the prizes, so that's £10,000 smackaroos minus a very few quid in costs every day to GMTV's bottom line. Not at all bad for three minutes of airtime that you'd otherwise have had to fill with something interesting.

I mentioned that sometimes they're not giving away cars or holidays or villas; sometimes they're giving away £10,000 in cash. And what happens is that if you answered the question correctly yesterday, there's a chance that none other than Keith Chegwin is going to knock on your door, live during the programme, mind you, and hand over the wedge of money on-air.

Yes, that's right. Keith Chegwin – the bloke who did the quiz show for Channel Five with no clothes on. Total eejit.

So this would put you into a dilemma, wouldn't it? Most people wouldn't mind £10,000 in tax-free readies landing in their lap without very much effort; but ask yourself this. Would you really be willing to have Keith Chegwin knock on your door, which you have to answer in your PJs, and have him – laughing and burbling like an epileptic frog – and his camera crew bundle into your house first thing in the morning to give it to you? Would you?

Keep in mind that not only do you have the humiliation of having Keith Chegwin and a couple of million people in your house while you're looking and feeling your worst – you're also revealing to the nation that you are fat-headed enough to have entered a competition where the question is to name the present Queen of England, or something equally inane.

Ten thousand pounds in cash on one hand – national humiliation on the other. Ten thousand pounds versus being a laughing stock to your friends and family for years to come.

When the question this morning was an unusually difficult one – how many corners in a triangle or something – Lizzie asked me which one I'd choose: £10,000 and a visit from Keith or not. My reply was simple. I'd save up to give GMTV £10,000 in cash rather than have Keith Chegwin knock on my door. And if he did, I'd take a baseball bat to him. She decided on balance it was probably better not to enter the competition.

21 APRIL

Matt says he wants to go to Prague for the weekend with his mates, and my wife wants me to stop him. She's read all the articles in the Sunday supplements about Prague being the stag-party capital of Europe, with more hookers per square inch than the red-light district of Amsterdam. She doesn't quite put it like this, but the truth is that she's concerned about giving up 'her little boy' to the tender mercies of these dreadful women. All I'm thinking is, 'Good for you, son,' but obviously can't say it.

'He's 17,' I say, trying to give the impression that I'm as concerned as she is. 'I don't think we can stop him.' She looks sad. She knows I'm right, but she doesn't want me to be.

22 APRIL

The poor sods presenting the early evening news in ITV's super-galactic new set look more and more uncomfortable. This is not least because the bloke is about 18 inches taller than the woman. So the director has taken to standing her a few feet in front of him, which looks preposterous. If you haven't noticed it before, you will now.

24 APRIL

Urgh! My wife has been into the travel agents to ask about holidays. It seems that she told them we wanted to go somewhere not too far away, but where you could rely on good weather later in the year. Since the kids have grown up, we've always been sure to take our holidays during term-time and in winter. Well, the prices are lower and you've less chance of having other people's screaming brats around your feet. Anyway, apparently the women in the shop were very helpful and are sorting out some brochures. Oh good, a few evenings to look forward to of looking through holiday brochures. Excellent.

27 APRIL

It seems that Matt doesn't want to go to Prague after all. Are we relieved? No, I don't think so. He and his mates have decided to go away for a month in the summer instead – to Bangkok.

28 APRIL

Yet another item on what the BBC laughingly refers to as the 'news' about so-called binge-drinking among the young. It's an excuse to go out on the town with the cameras after chucking-out time to discover that it ought to be renamed chucking-up time. The streets are lined with hordes of young people, drunk as skunks, rolling out of pubs, staggering down pavements, the girls laughing and showing their tits to the camera, the blokes mostly looking for a fight.

Occasionally you also get to see one; some totally vile, beyond-description, out-of-his-tree arse-head arguing with another young bloke, often almost equally vile but slightly less able to look after himself.

Then you see it – the lashing fists and the flaying boots – usually more than one or two blokes on to a single victim, punching and kicking him as he falls on the floor, and then stamping on his head.

What do you think when you see this? Because, to be honest, this is the sort of stuff that makes me grumpier than almost anything else. What is going through the heads of these bloody louts to make them think this is a good idea? How can it possibly be their idea of a good time?

This is all a bit more serious than I know we're meant to be, but you really do despair, don't you? What would you say to those guys if you had the chance to talk to them? 'Do you realize you could have killed this bloke and spent the next 15 years in prison?' But if you did get the chance to say something as naive as that, you'd be sure the reply would be, 'Yeah, well, he had it coming, didn't he?' or, more probably, 'He dissed me.'

Anyway, the slightly lighter side of this phenomenon involves the young women. Recent reports have concentrated on how women are now drinking more heavily than men, and are making binge-drinking the object of their evening out.

The TV reporter goes out with a group of girls – usually but not necessarily from Newcastle or somewhere 'up north'. They're always noisy, usually fat, almost inevitably showing far more of their cleavage than anyone could possibly want to see, and sporting tiny skirts, ill-becoming hairstyles in various colours and the odd tattoo. Then we are treated to a shot of one of them putting away a pint alongside some idiot boy. Yes, that's right, with an action that at first makes you think she's thrown the pint over her shoulder, she's finished hers and is wiping her mouth with the back of her hand while he's still struggling. Then another. Then a row of 'shots'. Then something else with a name out of the weather forecast.

Later we see the girls out on the street, one of them usually lying on the ground or sitting – legs wide apart – head in hands. Meanwhile, several friends are standing nearby and fanning her.

Felix Dexter referred to this in our *Grumpy Old Men at Christmas* (available on DVD at all good stores). He said he could never work out what this fanning is for. Is it some new medical treatment? Some miracle cure for alcohol poisoning? A draft of air? I've also noticed that a variation of it seems to be applied in an effort to stop women from crying. How does that work exactly?

Anyway, where were we? Oh, yes. I'm not sure why it should be so noteworthy that women are drinking as much or more than men. They're doing the same amount of just about everything else that men used to do more of, so why not?

The Grumpy Old Man answer is that it's repulsive. Not that it's any better that young men should drink too much and fight and make total plonkers of themselves. It's just that women are in most ways the more sensible sex, so you'd hope they'd know better. And it's depressing and grump-making to see that apparently they don't.

30 APRIL

A note from Matt on the breakfast table this morning next to his empty bowl of cereal: 'Back tomorrow'. Well, you know, it's nice to have some information.

May

1 MAY

Do you sometimes wonder if you have accidentally pressed the magic button on your car that makes it invisible? I've had one of those days today, where you're driving along and people are walking out into the road in front of you, or pulling out of side turnings when you're hurtling towards them, just as though you're totally invisible.

I find this usually happens on Sundays, when all the people too ditsy or fat-headed to take their cars out the rest of the week take them for a spin or go to visit the aged auntie. However, sometimes, for no obvious reason, they all seem to be out on a weekday. Which is what happened today.

You have to admit that there is a fairly wide variety of totally cretinous behaviour exhibited by other drivers, and one of my favourites among them is what I call the 'I wonder what this is for?' syndrome. This is usually exemplified by the person 500 yards ahead of you who starts indicating to turn left. You're thinking that he's bound to have turned left well before you catch up with him, so you don't really bother to brake. Now the distance is only 300 yards, and funnily enough he's still showing no sign of turning off left. As you get ever closer, it becomes apparent that he doesn't know where the turning is, and is examining every driveway or lay-by on the off-chance that it's where they are going to lunch at Auntie Beryl's.

So eventually you have to brake hard, and now you're right behind him and you're both moving along at a crawl. Even from your vantage point behind his vehicle, you can see that there's no left turn for half a mile ahead, and eventually he sees it too and knocks off the indicator. He then speeds up a bit, but of course he's still looking for the turning and after another half a mile he starts indicating again. He slows down. You slow down. The left turn is approaching. Nearer, nearer, nearer.

And this is what I call the 'I wonder what this is for?' moment. Yes, that's right, if you start to turn that big round thing in front of you, you'll find that the car will turn at the same time. The bloke has slowed more or less to walking pace, and then starts to turn the steering wheel as though he's doing it for the first time ever. And in my by now fevered mind, I imagine him saying, 'Oh, look, that's interesting, if I turn this big round thing to the left, the car turns in the same direction.'

Just get the hell out of my sodding way and let me get on with the day!

'What I hate though is people who beep you when you're driving. You stop somewhere, and presumably you've stopped there for a reason. But there's always some dickhead who decides you're just taking in the view. And so he beeps you and that really gets me. Because what are you supposed to do? Where are you supposed to go? It's not a holiday, you're not relaxing, it's not the beach. You're trying to get somewhere ... obviously something's in the way. But the dick behind you thinks, "No, no, he's just hanging around." I usually jump out of the car and go,

"What? What? Come on, what?" And if they're too big
I go, "OK", and get back in again.'

DON WARRINGTON

3 MAY

News today of another 'gangland slaying'. It's odd that, isn't it?
There isn't a lot of call for the word 'slaying' in everyday life.
I always think that slaying is usually about St George and all
that stuff. Where do they get this shit from? John Stapleton told
me another good one today. 'Sneak preview'. He says there's no
such thing as a 'preview' any more. It's always got to be a 'sneak
preview'. 'But it isn't,' he says. 'The film company shot a trailer
at huge expense and sent it to us.' He says he always tries to
excise 'sneak' from his script, but I think I've noticed a few
sneaking through.

4 MAY

Very unusually for me, I sat up to the small hours yesterday
because I'd agreed to take part in a phone-in on ABC Radio in
Australia. They've been running the first series of *Grumpy Old
Men*, and wanted to discover if the phenomenon is international. Turns out it is – they had hundreds of calls.

Most of them were talking about the same stuff as us.
But here's the amazing thing; one of the callers said that what
irritated him was the 'upswing' people use at the end of
sentences as if everything is a question. It's something that was
identified by several of our own grumpies as driving them close
to distraction, and at the time we blamed the Australians,
especially the soaps. Well, it seems that Australians blame the
Australian soaps as well, and grumpies in Australia are as
irritated by it as we are.

The other thing someone said that convinced me they'd 'got it' was that they're irritated by the various pronunciations of 'Australia'. It seems that the least worst variation involves extra emphasis on the first syllable – AUS-tralia – however the one that makes them want to reach for an axe is when people miss out the first syllable altogether – 'Stralia.

But the example I enjoyed best – from a quintessentially Grumpy Old Man somewhere in Queensland I believe, was one I hadn't thought of at all. 'Essential oils'. This bloke was driven potty by references to 'essential oils' which are, self-evidently, not essential at all. He proposed renaming them 'optional oils' or 'discretionary oils'. Oils you can perfectly easily do without.

Just that alone made it worthwhile for me to stay up till 1 a.m.

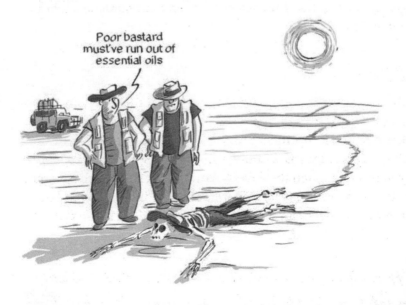

5 MAY

Do you remember when 'living statues' were good?

You know the sort of thing; bloke dressed as a Greek marble

statue or an extra from *Star Wars* standing stock-still. He'd have brilliant make-up, somehow manage to stay in one spot without twitching or moving a muscle for long periods, and then, just as a few people were wondering if he was real or not, he'd suddenly move and give the kids who'd ventured too close a terrible shock and the old ladies an involuntary shit.

I thought they were fun.

However, today I walked down that street from the Tube station to Covent Garden market and passed eight of them, and they were all bloody useless. A bloke I recognized as someone who until recently sold copies of the *Big Issue* was now sprayed silver. A man with almost as many spare tyres as me was pretending to be a Greek god. A bloke in a cardboard and tin-foil outfit made in his child's crèche was pretending to be a robot. All just shit.

8 MAY

After the conversation with John Stapleton the other day I guess I'm now highly sensitized to the use of preposterous words on the news. This morning I heard someone describe Harold Shipman's crimes as 'a killing spree'. Now 'spree' is not a word you hear that often these days – but I'd associate it with spending, a theme park or maybe even a drunken or drug-induced state. But the murder of an estimated 400 women? Let's think of another word, shall we?

'How about safety matches? I never get that. What is a safety match? What does that mean? It's a box of matches you could ignite; you could burn a house down.'

NIGEL HAVERS

12 MAY

Does anyone have any idea how the bastards managed to persuade us to drink water out of a bottle? It's a good one, isn't it? That's crept up on us over the years almost without us noticing it. Unless, of course, you're a grumpy, in which case it's been getting on your nerve endings for years.

When we were kids, we drank water out of a tap – day in, day out. And if you were lucky you got to put a bit of orange squash in it, or lemon barley if you came from a posh family. For a treat you might have a weekly bottle of R. White's Lemonade or Cream Soda. For the really decadent there might have been a bottle of Dandelion and Burdock, which now sounds like a class C drug.

If we were ever lucky enough to go abroad for our holidays, a major preoccupation was 'Can you drink the water?' I think we regarded whether you could or couldn't drink what came out of the local taps as a litmus test of the level of civilization. When I was 14, I went with my mum and dad to Venice, where it absolutely stank to high heaven, and we all came back with dysentery. 'Well, what do you expect?' asked my grandparents. Oh yes, you can tell that we were very cosmopolitan in our family.

So how did bottled water catch on here? I have an idea that it started with Perrier, which was a slightly less embarrassing way of saying 'I don't want a drink' when you went into a pub. If everyone else was having a pint or a glass of wine, and you didn't really want one, you felt better asking for a Perrier because at least it meant that you had a glass in your hand and you were paying to be there. And anyway, drinking water and having it come out of your nose was a bit of a novelty. Believe it or not, I think it probably seemed quite cool, for a nanosecond, to drink Perrier.

Then I seem to remember that maybe there were a couple of scares or doubts about tap water. Anyway, we somehow got it into our heads that drinking water out of a bottle was healthier than drinking it out of the tap. A new category and loads of shelf space needed for it at the supermarket. Suddenly the shopping trolley started getting laden down with huge six-packs of bottled water that you had to make a separate journey with to the car.

So did we get a discount off our water rates now we weren't drinking it? Quite the reverse. As the water companies were privatized (just one aspect of Mrs Thatcher's lunacy), our water rates went through the roof – all around the same time that we stopped drinking it from the tap. Well done, fellas.

I'm sure I then started seeing articles indicating that tap water is, in general, more pure than bottled water. So we've now come to a point where we are paying an arm and a leg to the water companies who are producing water that is purer and healthier than the water you'd buy in a bottle, yet we're still also buying it in a bottle.

I tried to persuade my family that this was senseless, and indeed started drinking tap water myself. I couldn't persuade anyone else to do this because, of course, water out of the tap isn't cold, so it doesn't taste as good as bottled water from the fridge.

So – and when they read this it will be the first time they know of it – I started filling up the bottles of water in the fridge with tap water to see if anyone noticed the difference. Needless to say, they didn't.

I don't think I could be bothered to maintain this lunatic regime for more than about three days, but it was long enough to prove my point. To myself at least.

So I'm happy to report that in my household … No, of course we haven't stopped. We still all drink water from a bottle because like just about everyone else out there, we're idiots with more money than common sense. We'd rather be made fools of by a brilliant marketing coup than be made to feel mean or eccentric by our loved ones.

'That never ceases to amaze me as well. You buy the bottle and it says that this water has been slowly formed over millions of years by the crustaceans or the volcanic rock ... through two ice ages and a stone age ... it is 80 million years old ... And then they bottle it all, and on the back is says "Use by September 05". It's just preposterous.'

RICK WAKEMAN

14 MAY

Just caught a story on the London 'News' Network that began 'Mayor Ken Livingstone will be grilled today by Conservatives ... ' And I guarantee that every single Grumpy Old Man within earshot said a version of the same thing: 'Oh really? Do we get to decide how high the flame is?'

16 MAY

Today is a very special day because I think it's the first day of the year so far that I have not felt grumpy for most or all of the day. That's because it's Sunday and because for once there has been nothing whatsoever that I have to do.

Do you remember Sundays when we were kids? Even though it was a day off school, I absolutely bloody hated Sundays, for the very reason that occasionally I like them now. Because there was sod all to do.

But the definition of 'sod all to do' then was very different indeed from what it is today. Oh, yes. When we said 'sod all to do' in those days, we really meant it.

It meant no telly, no iPod, no CDs, no DVDs, no computer

games, no shops open, no playing outside in the street. Worse even than that – for my brother and me it meant putting on our best clothes, waiting for what seemed like hours in the drizzle for the number 2 bus to take us up to Crystal Palace, and sitting talking to my grandmother for what seemed like a quarter of my total life-span. Eventually my mum and dad would come to collect us, but could we go home even then? Could we hell. We'd have to sit quietly for another millennium while they chatted about the various vastly important things that had happened since they'd last spoken three days ago. Like the milkman had left a bottle of silver top instead of gold. And all the while my brother and I had to be on our best behaviour on pain of a protracted and violent death. Finally, we'd be taken home, change out of our best clothes, have lunch (which in those days we called dinner), wash and dry the dishes (which in the pre-Teflon days took three hours), and then have to sit or play quietly while my parents watched Liberace on the telly.

Liberace. Can you believe it? A fat poof with a spangly jacket and bouffant hairdo, a grand piano and candelabra. Were we sophisticated or what?

Wow, even as I recall it, I wince to think how shit that used to be.

Nowadays on a Sunday you can do just about everything you might want to do on a weekday – get the bus, go to the pictures, go shopping, go bowling if you're potty enough, and no doubt you can even go to a lap-dancing club. Naturally enough, now that I can do any of those things, I don't want to. The idea of going shopping or bowling on a Sunday fills me with nearly as much dread as listening to Liberace did when I was 12.

When I was 12 I would have wanted to be able to do all the things I now can do aged 53. Now that I'm 53, I'd really like my Sundays to be like they were when I was 12. I suppose that's what's called a grumpy disposition.

19 MAY

I think I forgot to mention that, in a moment of madness, I've sent off to one of the TV shopping channels for one of those multi-gyms. Yes I know, I know – what happened to the membership of Piss-Pots? Well, I just reckon that if the kit is actually in my house, I'm much more likely to use it. That's the theory anyway. So, a bloody great big carton arrived today when I was out, and apparently the guy delivering it asked if we'd arranged for someone to come and assemble it. As I'd neglected even to tell the wife that I was sending for this item, she was unable to answer. Apparently the man looked sympathetic and left the box in the garage.

Anyway the 'handy flat-pack', thus described by the suntanned and finely honed presenter, turned out to be the size of Joan Collins' wardrobe and a little heavier. Decided to wait till the weekend to tackle it.

20 MAY

Don't you just love it when someone tells you they've actually spent the last few years hating something that you've thought they've been pleased with?

Today my wife decided to tell me that she has never really been pleased with the car she's driving. It's a VW Polo. She's had it for three years, and I distinctly remember a whole series of discussions about how good it is. Easy to park. Nippy around town. Economical. Reliable. With all these attributes, I've been assuming all this time that we liked the car.

But no, apparently it's only me who's liked the car. My wife has always felt that it 'lacks power'.

Of all its many wonderful features, I have to confess that having available great surges of power is not one that I would have attributed to this car, but still I'm a bit amazed. It trundles along fairly comfortably at 80 mph on the motorway. What do we expect it to do – win the Le Mans 24-hour race?

'There's nothing under the bonnet if you need to get away fast.'

Nothing under the bonnet? Nothing under the bonnet? Now I'm wondering when did my wife suddenly start sounding like Jeremy Clarkson? Ten minutes ago she thought a bonnet was something you wore at Easter.

At this point I know it's available to me to change the subject; and, indeed, the subject might go away for weeks or even months. The trouble now is that it's 'out there'. Any vague enjoyment I might ever have had of being in the car is now always going to be slightly overlaid by my knowledge that my wife doesn't really like it.

If we're on the motorway and wanting to overtake, I'm going to feel obliged to whack up the revs to show that we can indeed get past that milk float on the inside lane. As we start up a steep hill, I'm going to be changing down a gear rather sooner so we don't start to labour before we get to the brow. I know that, maybe not this week, and maybe not next week, but sooner or later I'm going to have to get a new and more powerful car.

It's not that I don't want a new car. It's not even that I wouldn't like a new car. As with everything else, it's just all the bollocks that you have to go through to swap this car for that.

Yes, that'll be another major irritant to look forward to in the weeks ahead.

22 MAY

Spent the afternoon lying flat on my back. Having a nice rest, you might be thinking. No, in agony from having twisted something while trying to assemble the multi-gym.

Yes, go on, go ahead and take the piss. The whole thing was the definition of the archetypal self-assembly nightmare. About a thousand pieces, none of them immediately identifiable as having anything in common with the diagram, which covered six pages and looked like the instructions on how to make a nuclear bomb. Except more technical. And obscure. There were about 300 bolts, of four different sizes, but with only a few millimetres differentiating each type. So naturally you're going to use the wrong one for the wrong thing, and end up having to disassemble the various bits you've put together – upside down.

Inevitably, in order to attach sprocket C to flange F, you have to reach across the parts you've already assembled at an awkward angle and that's when I felt something go in my back like a piece of snapping piano wire. That's what it felt like, and that's what it sounded like as well.

Excellent. A great start to my new exercise regime. The multi-gym is half-assembled in the garage, and I'm unlikely to be able to move comfortably for a week.

29 MAY

So guess what I did today? Yes, that's right; I went out to prospect the idea of buying a new car. We've established that there are many things about the Polo that my wife likes, and yes, she would like another VW, but maybe something with a bit more 'oomph'. I suppose I should be grateful that she's not asking for more 'va va voom'.

Of course, the local VW garage from which we bought the Polo closed down about a month after the purchase – thereby negating one of the main reasons why we chose VW. That means the next nearest VW garage is in Battersea, so, as it's the weekend and most people are off work, we get to sit in a long traffic queue. That's what I want to do on my day off. The journey is about 6 miles, so it takes about an hour to get there, and my back is still stiff, so already I'm in the best of moods by the time I enter the showroom.

Of all the 'bloke' things you sort of have to do, buying a car counts among the ones I hate most. On the whole I don't like the kind of men you have to deal with when you're buying something like this. I don't like being pissed about and asked if I want a cup of tea while I wait, and I don't like the feeling of being 'handled'.

Do you know what I mean?

'Are we looking for a new car or maybe a pre-owned?' 'Pre-owned' is what they now call what was once called 'second-hand'. This is the motoring equivalent of television's 'a second chance to see'.

'I'm not sure what *you're* looking for [I know I shouldn't do this, but truly, I just cannot help myself], but *I'm* probably looking for a new one. I've got a used one already.'

'And are we thinking of trading that in, or maybe of a private sale?' He still hasn't got it, and already I'm beaten down.

'We're thinking of a trade-in.'

'And would we be paying cash or wanting finance?'

'Well, at the moment I'm just thinking of buying a new car, and I'd like to see some.'

Now, I know that these guys have been trained, like any salesmen, to do the deal there and then. They've been told that if they let you out of the showroom, you'll probably never come back, so they want to get you committed as quickly as possible.

'Yes, I see. And if we can agree terms, are you ready to do a deal today?'

By now I've had it. I'm being 'handled'.

'Can we look at some cars?'

Apparently that's 'No trouble at all, sir.' And apparently, 'That's why we're here,' which is a revelation in itself.

We then go through all the variations – from sporty

two-door coupés, via the rather more sedate (but elegant) saloons, to the 4 x 4s. We go through engine sizes, types of metallic paint, upholstery and CD changers. There are optional cruise controls, GPS systems and cup-holders, various.

Not until he finally draws breath do I get the chance to say the thing I've been trying to say since I got here. 'Actually, I rather wanted one like the one we've got at the moment, except more powerful.' And even as I say it, I know that the moment has passed. When I came into this showroom I was ready to get a valuation on my car, sign a cheque and walk out having done the deal on the new car. Now I know that nothing will persuade me to buy a car from this bloke. Nothing. Because I'm fed up. The tide has gone out; the moment has gone.

The trouble is that this is the only VW garage for miles around, and I know that eventually I'm going to have to come back and go through this awful palaver again – from scratch. But at this moment I just cannot get out of the place fast enough.

I see that he is genuinely nonplussed when I tell him that I've run out of time and have to go. He was on a roll. Reckoned I was a dead cert.

For a moment I feel bad for him and want to say, 'Not your fault, mate, it's me.' But then I think 'What the hell', and head off home for my tea.

30 MAY

Heard a report from the Congo on the World Service this morning. The reporter was venturing out of the capital, Goma, in her car. 'It's too dangerous to venture far away from the city,' she said, 'so I turn the car around. To turn a whole nation around will be much harder.' What, turning the nation around is even harder than turning a car around? Extraordinary.

31 MAY

It seems to me that religion is one thing and the Church is quite another, neither of which we want to spend a lot of time talking about here. But you've really got to wonder, haven't you, what on earth anyone thinks is going on in the Church of England?

Today the papers are full of all the stories they are full of every day: new record number of reported rape cases, new low in conviction rates; it seems that we've forgotten the people of the Sudan, who were all the rage just a few months ago, and thousands of them are starving; we've got anti-Semitism, jihads in our streets, unprecedented violent crime, and that's not to mention more coveting of thy neighbour's wife and ox than in the longest time. And what are these C of E guys getting themselves into a state about? Where the gay ones put their willies.

Yep, that's it. The latest development in the seemingly everlasting saga of schism or excommunication or consignment to eternal hellfire and damnation. The American and Canadian churches have been told to go and stand in the corner and not show their faces or their dirty little hands until they've scrubbed out their mouths with carbolic.

I used to know a few people in the Church and they were relatively sensible people. God knows who's running it now (or at least we hope so), but how these guys can think it's OK to be preoccupied with something as pitifully trivial as gay bishops – which every sane person got over years ago – when the world is going to hell faster than a speeding rocket, leaves you gasping. Doesn't it?

June

2 JUNE

I made the same mistake today that I've been making all too frequently recently, and found myself in one of those vast and dreadful electrical superstore places trying to buy a new telly. I have wittered on at great length before about how electrical 'superstores' never have the item in stock that you choose from the display, so I won't do it again. Suffice it to say that this is what happened today.

However, during the inevitable tortured process of determining that they didn't have any of the items I wanted, I witnessed a woman trying to buy a new telly because, she said, her existing one couldn't receive Channel 5, or 'five', as it now prefers to be called.

'Will this one be able to get Channel 5?' she asked the assistant.

I was just about to intervene and say that if her current telly didn't receive Channel 5, it was more likely to be about the aerial, or the place she lives in than the telly, but then I thought, 'Hey, what's it got to do with me?' Anyway, he was well on the case:

'Yes,' he said confidently, 'all five channels, or we can sell you a satellite system that will give you 300 or more channels.'

'Oh no, I just want to add Channel 5. My nephew sometimes comes to visit and he likes to watch it. I said I'd get it for him next time he comes around.'

My instinct was to ask her whether it was wise to provide her nephew with Channel 5 just because he wanted it, but I know from experience that these interventions can be taken the wrong way. Anyway the assistant goes ahead and sells her a horrible new telly with loads of gizmos she doesn't want or need, and then he starts.

'Can I interest you in the extended warranty, which covers you for parts and labour for up to three years? It's only £80 and it'll give you a replacement set if anything happens to this one in that time.'

She catches my eye at this point and I can't stop myself. I shake my head – but she obviously thinks I'm some kind of pervert or care-in-the-community case because she looks away and says to the assistant, 'Oh well, I'll probably have lost it by the time I need a repair, but go on then.'

You'd think he'd quit while he was ahead, but he hasn't finished.

'Well, since you've made that wise decision, I wonder if you'd like to extend it to a five-year guarantee for just another £20?' She looks at me again, and this time I do my level best not to look deranged, and again I shake my head. I don't know if it was anything to do with me, but now even she seems to have had enough.

'No, no, I only came out because I wanted Channel 5. I think this is probably enough now.'

'How about if I give it to you for an extra £10?'

'Oh, go on then ... ' she's weakened. She's going to pay an extra £90 – more than half the cost of the telly, for a guarantee she'll never ever use.

Since I am not quite deranged enough to tell her in the shop, let's put it on the record now. Extended warranties are a rip-off. You get at least a 12-month guarantee from the manufacturer, sometimes more. If your appliance breaks down after that, you are a) very unlikely to remember that you bought an extended warranty in the first place; b) if you do remember, very unlikely to be able to find it; c) one of the very few things that has improved in recent years is the reliability of electrical goods: short of built-in obsolescence they very rarely break down; and d) by the time you've had the appliance sent back to the shop, been pissed about, they don't have the parts, it has to be sent off, etc., etc., etc., you'd be better off buying a new one anyway.

One of the leading electrical hardware shops recently made nearly as much money from extended warranties as from selling the products. Don't buy them. Just tell the slug in the shop that you are a Grumpy Old Man. That ought to abbreviate the process.

'I bought a television set not so long ago and the guy who was putting in the television realized that there was something wrong with the aerial, so we had to have an aerial man then. They had a discussion and they were asking me questions about it, and I don't know anything about it at all. I mean the fact that you work in television doesn't mean you know anything about televisions. So this debate went on and on about where the aerial should be. Was there one on the roof? How do I know? Have I been on the roof? It's just, "Look, I want a television and I want to be able to turn it on and I want those channels. Over to you, pally. Don't keep asking me questions about the damn thing."'

DES LYNAM

4 JUNE

On reviewing recent entries into this bilious journal, I've had an idea that could make life so much easier for so many Grumpy Old Men, and for so many of the people who have to deal with us and generally put up with us on a daily basis.

We should carry an identity card.

In the 1980s I carried in my wallet, next to my 'Switch me off if I'm a vegetable' card, a little plastic card that said something like 'In the event that I should be the victim of a major disaster and unable to express my own wishes, this is to certify that I do not wish to be visited by Mrs Thatcher.' It was during the time that she kept on mawkishly turning up at the bedsides of victims of ferry disasters or major fires, complete with television cameras, doing her very strange 'angel of mercy' act. Can you imagine anything worse? No, really think about it. Already you're the victim of a terrible arbitrary tragedy. Your life has gone to hell; you're halfway comatose, and finally you come round to find Mrs Thatcher dribbling over you and looking concerned in front of 150 cameras. You'd immediately believe that you'd died and gone to hell. At the very least, you'd certainly have to wonder what terrible thing you'd done in an earlier life to deserve that, now wouldn't you?

But that's a bit of a diversion. The card I have in mind would be the equivalent of carrying a card saying that you are profoundly deaf, in the hope that it would stop people trying to sell you an iPod; or a card saying that you are a vegetarian in case someone tries to force-feed you a pork chop. Not that frequent an occurrence, but you probably get the idea.

If you had a card explaining in the clearest and most straightforward possible terms that you are a Grumpy Old Man, it would simply mean that no one should try to sell you a load of old bollocks of any description. It would save so much time and embarrassment.

In my case, in recent weeks it would have saved me having to explain to the poor sod who was trying to sell me a VW that my patience quota had expired for the day and I had to get home. In electrical stores it would mean salesmen wouldn't try to sell you the extended warranty. As you hurry through the ground floor of department stores, you could hold up the card and you would immediately cut a swathe through those absolutely appalling women who lurk on all sides wearing what I assume are Hallowe'en masks, even though it isn't All Hallows Eve, and ask you if you'd like to stop for a moment to try a whiff of this new 'fragrance for men'.

Better still, we might be able to have it as a little monogram on a collar or, for more formal occasions, on a tie. GOM. A little piece of shorthand that would save so much time and bollocks. What do you think? Do we have a national movement?

6 JUNE

Managed to assemble the rest of the multi-gym today. I finished it off in the garage, and only then did I realize that it was too big to go through the various doors into the spare room where I plan to keep it. Wonderful. Therefore had to strategically disassemble it. By the end of the day it was up and apparently working, but of course I was too knackered to try it out.

9 JUNE

One of the many reasons why I'm grumpy is that I'm constantly answering the phone and it's never for me. I'm not complaining that the call is never for me; the very last thing I want is people calling me up at home for any reason, and I always breathe a slight sigh of relief when the caller asks for the wife or one of the kids. Except that I then have to walk all around the house trying to track them down, and bellowing over the deafening sound of some awful 'music'.

Actually, it's rather surprising that the phone rings as often as it does. I say that partly because the wife and kids all have mobiles, but more because I'm told that the kids' friends hate it when I answer the phone. Apparently I'm brusque.

Actually 'brusque' is probably a very good word for what I am on the telephone, but I genuinely don't think I can work out what the problem is.

I'll freely admit that I've certainly never been one of those dads who answers with a cheery variation of 'Battersea Dogs' Home', or asks 'Who's speaking?' and then goes on to ask Zoe or Paul or whichever friend it is how they are, how their parents are, that I hope they are revising harder than Matt or Lizzie, and did they enjoy their holiday. I can't imagine anything worse, if you're a 17-year-old, than having your life interrupted by some old fart apparently trying to find some common ground with you, when all you want them to do is to go off and die and leave you a handsome inheritance.

No, I answer the phone with the word 'Hello', which seems uncontroversial. I listen as carefully as I can, and then say 'I'll get him/her.' I then go about the house room by room, searching or following the strains of Robbie Williams as they echo across the landing and down the stairs.

I've made a few attempts over the years to persuade the kids to answer the phone because nine times out of ten the call is for them. Making no headway at all, and eventually exasperated, I once tried a different approach. I'd answer the phone, ascertain that the call was for one of the kids, and then leave the receiver lying on the table beside the phone and get back to whatever I was doing. I worked out that the friends would find this so frustrating that they'd persuade my kids to answer the phone quickly or, better still, stop calling. Needless to say, this course of action led to complaints of unreasonable behaviour, in which my wife rather disloyally concurred, and the practice had to be stopped.

'The other thing on the phone is people ring you up at home and offer to sell you things. You even get answer phones ringing you up and saying you've won a holiday in Disneyland. Piss off ... A friend of mine has done this and I'm gonna start doing it now, which is to say to the guy who rings you up, "I can't actually talk to you now – I'm a bit busy – but give me your home phone number and I'll ring you back tonight." And they go, "Oh, I'm not supposed to do that." "Well, you've just rung me at home. Just give us your number and I'll ring you at home tonight." Everyone do it!'

JOHN O'FARRELL

12 JUNE

You have to wonder, don't you, if there is any security guard, butler, footman (whatever that is) or court sodding jester working in any of the royal palaces or Parliament that isn't an undercover reporter for a tabloid newspaper? Yet another 'shocking breach' today that will leave us reeling, apparently. I think these editor guys have a mental picture of us all stopping strangers in the street and saying how shocking it is that our beloved Royal Family is so poorly protected. Well, actually I don't find that I do a lot of 'reeling' when I read that a news-paper journalist has conned his way into close proximity with

Prince Nobody or the home secretary. In fact, I don't think it even spoils my breakfast. I just think, 'For God's sake ... as though anyone cares!' and I strongly suspect that most other people think the same.

16 JUNE

'How's it going with the multi-gym?' my wife asked, rather sarcastically, I thought.

'I've bought it for all of us to use,' I said, 'not just me.'

'Yeah, right,' she said. I hate that, don't you?

18 JUNE

What about introducing a congestion charge for the Tube?

No really, think about it, and let's apply the rationale that led to the congestion charge on the roads.

Loads of people used to go to work in London in their cars. Some pointy-head reckoned there were too many; they were causing delays, everyone was getting bad-tempered, there were just far too many people doing it. So what did they think was the answer when supply exceeded demand? Make people pay more so that demand decreases.

There was every kind of joy among the bus-huggers in London when the congestion charge reduced the number of cars coming into London. Big surprise, huh? Charge people an extra £5 a day for doing something, and fewer of them will do it. Actually, I know a way of solving the traffic problem altogether. Charge £100 a day; there'll hardly be a vehicle on the roads. Take a bow.

However, that's not my point today. My point is that if a congestion charge is deemed appropriate when things are overcrowded, uncomfortable and causing delays, let's have one for the Tube. I went on the Tube today, on the Northern Line, and it was absolutely and unbelievably wall-to-wall and floor-to-ceiling packed.

First of all, the platform is total bloody mayhem. You are jammed in shoulder to shoulder and all the time you can see more people streaming in. If you are three or four rows back from the edge of the platform, you know you aren't going to get into the carriage. If you are at the front, you are in imminent peril of being shoved on to the track and squished in one of the most horrible deaths imaginable.

The train comes in, and even before it stops you can see it's packed to capacity with a seething mass of humanity. The doors slide open and none of the passengers makes the slightest effort to create space for people to get on. They're doing what we all do – hoping that the people on the platform would prefer to wait for the next train than to endure the experience of an over-familiar sardine.

I manage to get a toe-hold in the doorway, but, being of the taller persuasion, I stand in grave danger of decapitation once the doors slide shut. As they do so, I bow my head, and then am destined to stand in the shape of a banana; and at my age and with my back, that's not a good position. That's not to mention how much of a prat I feel.

This has to be endured for a couple of stops, and then I'm able to edge a bit further into the train. At this point I have my head stuck next to the sweaty armpit of a Scotsman who, I'm guessing, was seriously on the piss last night. I'm guessing this because it seems that his body is trying to expel about 18 pints before he gets to work. Oh, and before you say I'm being unfair and ask how I knew he was Scots, he had it tattooed across his forehead.

Sitting on the bench below me is a bloke with an MP3, which is blasting the most extraordinary din directly into his earholes. Now I swear that everyone in the carriage can hear this from up to 20 feet away. What the hell does it sound like when fed directly into your cranium? All we can hear is the cymbals. Over and over and over again. God only knows what *he's* hearing.

Next to him there's a bloke reading the *Telegraph* and getting more and more irritated that the bloke on the other side is conspicuously reading it over his shoulder. This is so obvious that I'm almost expecting the second bloke to ask him to wait for a minute before turning the page.

So just stand back and take an objective look at this scene. We're British, and thus predisposed to be reserved. We are not naturally a gregarious people; we like our own personal space, we don't like to sweat or get into a bad temper. Just stand back and take a really hard look at this pathetic mass of sentient beings crammed into a tiny underground tube of metal, all on their way to spend eight or nine hours in an office with overhead fluorescent lights, staring at a tiny computer screen, alongside people they don't really like, and then at the end of it they're going to do the same in reverse. All for not quite enough pay to meet all their weekly bills, so they've all got huge debts on their 15 credit cards. Day in day out, month in month out, year after year.

What is this like, eh? Last time I looked, we have only one life. One visit to this planet, just a few years to make the most of, to spend as we wish. One chance to make a mark, make a difference.

Keep that thought in mind next time you sit on the Northern Line. And get grumpy. Get really, really grumpy.

19 JUNE

Got home this evening to find the dining table covered in holiday brochures. Pages and pages and pages of glossy photographs of tower blocks by the sea, swimming pools in every shape and size, and promises of oodles of 'local colour'. My heart sank. The only upside is that there were brochures of everywhere from Spain to Bali, so I know that not much progress has been made in narrowing it down. The strategy lives to fight another day.

21 JUNE

Wimbledon. You have to wonder who to feel more sorry for, don't you? The crowds of fans who turn out pathetically every year to wave their flags and shake their booties in the hope that Tim Henman is at last going to achieve something fabulous, or Tim bloody stupid Henman himself.

By the time you read this, of course, it could be that I've been proven wrong and that he's the hero of the hour. But on the form of recent years, he's about as likely to win the Wimbledon tennis tournament as I am.

Poor old bugger. He's just the latest in a long line of British 'heroes' on whom we lamely pin our hopes. A triumph of hope over optimism. It's some sort of pathetic patriotic fervour that manages to blind us to what everyone else in the world can see perfectly clearly. We're crap. Like when the people of Manchester persuaded themselves a few years ago that they had a hope of winning the bid for the Olympic Games. I believe that was the time Atlanta eventually won it. Manchester – Atlanta? Manchester – Atlanta? A difficult one, eh? What were they thinking?

So poor old Tim Henman. A delightful bloke, no doubt, but just not a first-rate player, and carrying the hopes of the nation on his shoulders year after year. You can tell it in his face; even he doesn't think he has a prayer. But year after year thousands of idiots stand on that slope with the big screen watching his matches in the tournament and yelling 'Tim' as though he's a pop star. During the quarter-final, or wherever it is that he's eventually knocked out, some idiot in the crowd only has to yell 'Come on, Tim' and everyone erupts in adulatory cheers. Embarrassing for everyone concerned.

Tennis is only the latest in a long line of games that we British invented, got good at, but then made the mistake of teaching to the rest of the world. No sooner had everyone else learnt it than they got better than we are. It's happened with football, cricket, rugby and probably loads of other things. We're OK until the rest of the world 'gets it', and then they start beating us.

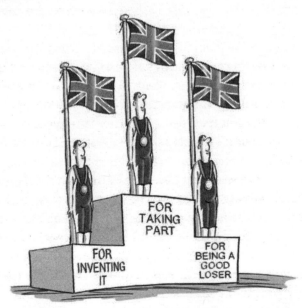

So that's why we need to start inventing lots of other sports that we can excel at for a few years before other people 'get it' – such as darts or synchronized swimming. No one actually thinks they're real sports, but maybe we can stay ahead of the game to win the odd event before the Africans start doing it and beat us hollow.

Or is that too cynical?

'I do feel sorry for Tim. It's like a recurring nightmare, isn't it? Every time he gets to this stage in Wimbledon you think, "God this must be a dream because I'm sure this has happened before." And it does, again and again and again and again and again, and he's not going to do it, is he? He's not going to do it.'

SIR GERRY ROBINSON

22 JUNE

One of the many enormous joys of descending into old-gitdom is that I find I've started to spill a lot of stuff down my front.

I noticed that my old father-in-law used to do this a lot, especially in the last few years of his life. Mind you, he was about 78, and I don't think his tendency started quite as early as mine has.

George was a wonderful bloke. 'Oh, bugger,' he'd say, immediately wiping the mustard or whatever it was off his tie, and thereby smearing it over a wider area and making the whole problem far more conspicuous. At least he always had the alternative of removing his tie. I, thank God, never have to wear a tie these days. However, the downside is that I've got no fall-back when the Pan-Yan or soy sauce slops liberally across my shirt or pullover. There's nowhere to hide.

I'm not sure what it is. I don't think I'm actually missing my mouth more. Maybe I'm just trying to get more in. Actually, if I'm honest, what I actually believe is that the wife is making increasingly sloppy sandwiches, with ingredients that are prone to falling out. However, I'm afraid that if I tell her, she'll stop making them at all.

On the following day it seems a bit much to have to put the pullover with the little smudge on the front through the wash for the sake of a tiny remnant of a stain, so I usually ignore it and wear the same thing again. So now I've become one of those senile and sad old sods who walks around with rubbed-in stains down his front, bits of missed whiskers sticking out under my nostrils or chin, worn and stained jeans and a jumper you could boil up and make soup.

I'll bet you wish you knew me better, don't you?

'Yeah, it does seem wrong to wash a pullover after only one or two outings. To me it's like seven, eight or even ten outings, so if you've got your sprouts or stuff down it … I'm not as bad as I used to be because in my smoking days my jumpers would be full of burnt holes as well as custard and stuff.'

ARTHUR SMITH

23 JUNE

For some time I've been exchanging emails with some bloke about a business proposition too boring to talk about, but today his PA called up and asked if she could book some 'face time' with me.

'Is that the expression he used?' I enquired.

'What?'

'Face time. Did he ask if you could book some face time?'

'Yes, I think so.'

As politely as I could, I declined. Can you imagine having to deal with someone who uses expressions like 'face time'?

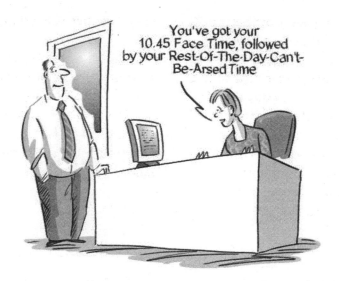

You've got your 10.45 Face Time, followed by your Rest-Of-The-Day-Can't-Be-Arsed Time

24 JUNE

How did it happen, do you suppose, that every time you turn on the telly these days, there's a bloke blubbing?

If it isn't Matthew Pinsent winning an Olympic medal, it's that effeminate-looking bloke with the dyed-blonde hair from the *X Factor*. You know, four Welsh lads, one of them was a bit tubby. Sang 'Bohemian Rhapsody' and all that. G Mex? G-string? Something or other.

Any time I had the misfortune to catch *Pop Idol* or whatever the latest clone was called, the blokes would break down in tears if they were 'coming to London'; they were hysterical if they weren't 'coming to London'; and most of them were in tears on the phone to their mums in between.

So this is interesting territory for Grumpy Old Men. Most of us were brought up by dads who had done military service. Maybe fought in the war. These guys actually had something to weep about, but very few of them did. Not in our presence anyway. We were brought up in a world where girls cried and men did not. Actually, I'm sure this is a very non-PC thing to say these days, but I think we thought that for boys to cry was a bit cissy. Certainly, if you did, you could expect to have the piss taken out of you by your mates for years.

We didn't see Clint Eastwood crying, did we? Or Gary Cooper? Not a lot of tears shed by Steve McQueen I recall, or Kirk Douglas.

No doubt that's our problem, and it must be healthy for blokes to get more in touch with their emotions. Do you think? But I just can't get used to it.

Matthew we can understand. Four years of busting your arse day in day out to try to live up to Sir Stephen Redgrave; you pull it off by a hair's breadth, and then realize it's all downhill from there. I guess you can forgive a bit of emotion. And anyway, who among us is going to imply that there's anything cissy about Matthew Pinsent?

But all these big babies with engineered jeans and high-lights; what are they all thinking of? Get a grip kids. Or at least save it for something that matters.

28 JUNE

It's funny, isn't it, how we can get used to things being called things that they obviously aren't?

The most obvious example is tea. I know I've gone on about this in relation to 'tea' in Starbucks before, but when we were kids a cup of tea was made by brewing tea leaves in boiling water and pouring it into a cup. (For full and frankly exhausting instructions on how to make tea properly, please see *Grumpy Old Men: The Official Handbook*). Anyway, for those less keen on homework, just think about that process, and then think about what happens when you push the button marked 'tea' on the automatic machine in your office. Water that has been in the machine for days, was last boiled six hours ago, and is now tepid, strains briefly through a small coffin-shaped container full of the dust that is swept up from the floor after proper tea leaves are processed. It then mixes with a powder that they call 'milk' but isn't anything like it, and drops down into a plastic cup. It's an odd tan colour with a bit of floating scum on top. Well, whatever you think of the stuff that comes out, it's not tea, is it?

'You know, I'm absolutely certain that there's an array of 47 buttons and whatever one you press you get the same stuff. It's another of those choice things, isn't it? Do you want this? Do you want that? You press this button or that button – you want it white, you want latte, you push it down and the same stuff comes out the bottom. And it all tastes bloody terrible. In a way it sums up life, doesn't it? You know, sums up life in the modern age.'

SIR GERRY ROBINSON

30 JUNE

Nasal hair. No, I'm not going to go on about it – except to say that it's started to grow. Ignoring it doesn't seem to be an option, and tugging at it makes my eyes water. So am I going to have to invest in one of those little pointy shavers that goes up your nose? Oh, God, no. Please, say it ain't so.

July

1 JULY

The weather so far this year has been uniformly awful. Week after week, we've been waiting for the summer to start, and week after week it's been cold and wet and miserable.

But today, literally out of the blue with no warning, it was hot. In an instant everyone was walking around dressed like extras from *Baywatch*. Like they had it all laid out on the bed, waiting for the first glimpse of the sun. Cutaway T-shirts, bikini tops and tiny shorts, sandals, shades on the head, the whole nine yards.

I used to like it when the weather turned hot, but that was probably because as a very young man I thought that getting a suntan would improve my chances with women. I can't say that it noticeably did, but anyway the delusion lasted me for a few years. Then, of course, there was the upside that in this weather, women wear very few clothes. Again, as a younger man, this was a bit of a kick.

Today I don't care about a suntan because we've all had the fear of God put into us about skin cancer, and anyway the only thing I feel when I lie out in the sun is sweaty. I can't say that I don't like looking at girls with very little on, but at my age this is sad. And anyway, the prospect of being labelled as a dirty old man is so repugnant that I'd rather not take the risk. So I don't.

So there we are; even the sunshine makes me grumpy.

3 JULY

When we were kids, there were 'things' and then there was 'fashion'.

'Things' were the ordinary stuff that you needed – like a kettle, a bike, a pen or a clock. 'Fashion' was the stuff that was more discretionary and had to be up to date.

For example when 'loons' were all the rage, you'd rather stay home and watch *Double Your Money* than go out wearing straight-legged jeans. The idea of wearing a T-shirt with a collar once grandad-vests became objects of desire was obviously never an option.

However, the important point is that there was a difference between them.

The difference was that while fashion moved on from time to time and obliged you not to look too much of a prat wearing Tuf Townies when everyone else was wearing Spanish Desert Boots, you kept your 'things' until they were worn out or broken. 'Things' were more or less built to last.

Mostly, when something did go wrong with a 'thing', you'd get it mended. Like your toaster. There used to be places that would repair your vacuum cleaner. In the unlikely event that something was beyond repair and needed to be replaced, it might be that the technology had moved on a bit and you'd buy something more up to date than the one you were replacing. You'd find that the electrical cord went into the base of the kettle rather than the actual kettle; sounds like a good idea – less plugging and unplugging of electrical sockets with wet hands, etc. Cool.

What we Grumpy Old Men find a bit difficult to get our heads around now, though, is that today *everything* is fashion. Everything. In the unlikely event that you find yourself talking to a younger person about the idea of buying something, using it and keeping it until it is useless, or indeed the thought of something actually getting better and more desirable with age, they'd look at you as though you were what you actually are. A throwback.

This has all come to me because today, after about ten days of begging, pleading, cajoling and eventually humiliating ourselves, a BT engineer came to the house to fix a problem with one of our phone sockets. I'd say he was about 35, this bloke, and when he saw the phone we use next to the bed, he actually burst out laughing. Dunno why. It's not like it's a black Bakelite device with a dial or anything: you don't have to wind it up, or tap the cradle and ask for the operator. It's green, plastic, with push button numbers and the handset on a cradle. You've seen them thousands of times, but he said he hadn't seen one for years. He said it was called a 'trim-phone' and he reckoned we might even be able to get money for it.

Now I'm at a loss here because the truth is that this bloody phone is the only one in the house that I actually know how to work. You pick up the receiver, dial the number, sometimes get through to the person you want to speak to, complete the call and put down the phone. Sure, you can't wander around the house while you're doing so, but I usually find I can manage to stay in one place for the duration of one of my average phone calls.

The other phones all around the house, bought against my better judgement, have multiple handsets that peep and buzz and light up; every button has a selection of functions written underneath it like 'OGM play' or 'mode' or 'conf'. I don't know how to set the answering machine, and, worse still, I don't know how to play the recorded messages. However, I also don't know how to stop the bloody thing from making a 'peeping' sound at one-minute intervals to indicate that there are unheard messages.

When I bought the system, and this is honestly true, I asked the guy in the shop for the simplest one they had on sale. Maybe he was having a laugh and sold me the most complex, but I really don't think so.

Anyway, now I look around the house and find that everything we own – everything – is out of date. So, the grumpy observation for today? There used to be 'things' and there was 'fashion'. Now there's just 'fashion'. Everything has to be replaced frequently – not because it's broken, not because it no longer does what you want it to do – just because it's old. Not unlike my good self really.

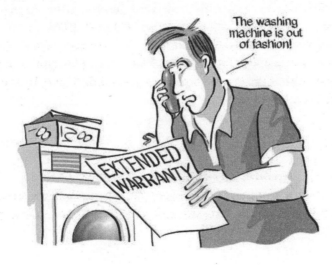

The washing machine is out of fashion!

6 JULY

Meal-deals. What on earth are they? Desperate for something to eat on the way home along the M3 today, I found myself queuing at the counter of Burger King. Even in these abstemious and cautious days, once in a while my better judgement will be suspended and I'll determine to eat something totally awful. I always regret it within five minutes, but for that five minutes it's just the thing I want.

Anyway I ordered a cheeseburger and fries, and the Bulgarian idiot behind the counter said:

'Vot drink d'you vont vith that?'

'I don't want a drink, thank you.'

'But it's a meal-deal. You got a free drink. You can haff Coke, Fanta, Sprite.'

So now I'm assuming that, though he says it's free, somewhere along the line I'm going to be charged for something I don't want, and am getting pissed off:

'But I didn't ask for a meal-deal. I just asked for a cheeseburger and fries.'

'Yiss, dot's a meal-deal. Free drink. Vont it or not?'

'If I'd wanted a sodding meal-deal, I'd have asked for it. Why do I have to speak your fucking stupid language, you squid-brain?' Of course I didn't say that. I thought it. But I didn't actually say it.

Meal-deals. What next?

8 JULY

Having reported only the other day that phone calls to the house are never for me, I had just got into the bath this evening when I heard the phone ringing and then Lizzie's voice saying 'I'll get him.'

'Who is it?'

'Dunno, they didn't say.'

I told Lizzie to tell them I'd ring back, but of course by then she was out of earshot.

Ordinarily, I would have just ignored it, but as I'd left six messages for the plumber this week and there was an off-chance he might return my call, I got out of the bath, put on my dressing-gown and hobbled, dripping liberally all over the hall carpet, to the phone.

'Hello?'

A voice I didn't recognize asked if it was me. I said that I presumed so.

'This is NatWest Bank. Would you mind if we asked you some questions?'

'Would I what?'

'It's NatWest Bank. Would you mind if I asked you some questions?'

Can you imagine? I was so apoplectic I just didn't know what to say. I felt like putting the phone down, getting dressed, driving to the nearest branch of NatWest and pissing through the letterbox. As it was, all I could do was to devastate him with my rapier-like wit.

'Yes, and if you ever ring here again I'll come down there, rip off your head and shit in it.'

'I tell them to piss off. I say, "Piss off, I haven't got time for this." Anyway, you haven't won anything, you know, they just want you to buy stuff. It is extraordinary that these people are cheerful when they ring you. They go, "Hello, how are you?" And you think, "I don't know you. Why are you talking to me as though I'm your best friend?" And I go, "Look, I'm really, really busy." And put the phone down. They say, "Is this a convenient moment?" And I go, "No", and they go, "When would be?" I say, "Well, six years' time. The summer of, I don't know, 2012 – that will be quite good. I'll be fine on a Wednesday afternoon."'

DON WARRINGTON

9 JULY

This morning a letter arrived from the Council Planning Department, and my heart sank as soon as I opened it. Our neighbours want to build an extension to their property. The council has determined that we are likely to be affected by this application and invites our comments. We are at liberty to view the plans at the local planning department between the hours of 9.30 a.m. and 5 p.m., Monday to Friday. We have 21 days to register our comments, and of course anything we say will be made public.

So that's just great, isn't it?

As with anything I get through the post from the council, all my instincts are to rip up the letter and toss it in the bin. But if I do that, the next thing I know will be that a tower block will be built just over the fence, with 150 balconies overlooking my pitifully tiny back garden. So now I've got to find time to drive into town, look for somewhere to park, ponce about seeking out the planning department, hang about while some air-head sorts out the plans – except that he'll be 'on lunch' – and then eventually, if and when I get to see them, I won't be able to make head or tail of them.

There is, of course, always an alternative. I can shrug my shoulders, resign myself to months of construction lorries, builders, mud, noise, dust, more mud, our foundations being undermined, after all of which our property will be worth £50,000 less than it is today. Or I can take the time and trouble to object, go through a long and unpleasant process, fall out with my neighbour, and in that instance I have to think of a reason to oppose the idea that sounds more legitimate than 'I just don't want it.' And it'll all end up the same anyway: he'll get permission and I'll be pissed off.

Excellent.

15 JULY

What is it about vandals that they all have blurred faces? It seems that three times a week there's a news item about vandalism, and every story is illustrated by bands of yobs with hoods, cycling by on BMX bikes, or jumping up and down on the windscreens of cars. And every time their faces have been obliterated by that process that I think is called 'pixelation' or something.

Why is that? When I was a trainee journalist, we learnt that you could not show a picture of someone who was the subject of court proceedings where identification might be an issue. But that doesn't seem to be the case with these guys. Here they are, usually aware that there is a camera present, smashing up someone else's property. They don't even care that we can see who they are.

So why disguise them? They're doing it. There can be no dispute. I'd vote that their faces should always be shown so that if we happen to recognize someone, we can be at liberty to go round to their house and lob a brick through the window. Or, if they are particularly young and we feel so inclined, we can give them a sharp smack across the top of the head if we see them at the shops.

Why are we disguising them? Fuck 'em.

'I think we should be able to buy a decoder that turns the pixelated faces back into their real ones so we should be able to identify them. And then, once we've identified them, they should be arrested and then have their faces pixelated for real. So when they walked around they actually had those pixelated faces, so we'd know who they were.'

RICK WAKEMAN

18 JULY

Do you ever wonder why hand-driers never work?

It can't be the most difficult piece of technology in the world, now can it? What I actually want in a men's room is hot and cold running water, a soap dispenser with soap in it, a paper towel and a waste-bin to put it in that isn't overflowing. However, I realize that's far too difficult, so I guess we have to make do with a machine that blows hot air. All we want out of this is something that turns on, either when you push a button at the side or when you put your hands where the blast should be; remains at a reasonable temperature, neither too hot nor too cold; and stays blowing for enough time for your hands to be dry. How hard can that be?

Well, how many variations of getting it wrong will you come across in an average week out and about? If switch-operated, the switch doesn't work. If automatic, it doesn't come on when you put your hands underneath. If the blast of air does come on, it's too hot, or too cold. *And it never stays on for enough time!*

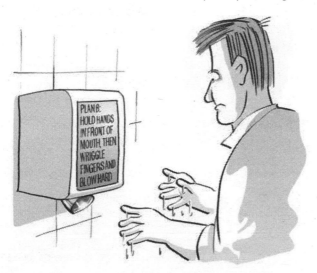

So you take your hands away and put them back again, hoping for a second blast. No such luck. Or you give up and leave the room, wiping your hands on your jeans.

I've now decided not to bother and I always leave the men's room with wet hands. Hell, they dry in a few minutes anyway. The only problem comes when you happen to run into someone you know outside the door and they want to shake hands with you. What you really don't want to do is to shake hands with someone who's just come out of the can and has wet hands. So, I find myself apologizing, explaining that the hand-driers don't work, and shaking my hands around like a girl trying to dry her nail polish.

Yep – just one more thing to get into our various crevices.

20 JULY

Do you remember when DVDs came out and people said that the great thing about them was that they couldn't get damaged? Yes, great new technology apparently. Of course, you'd have to replace everything you've collected on VHS over the years, but it'd be worth it because these would last for ever. I now find that every second DVD we rent from Blockbusters starts to piss about around two-thirds of the way through. The action stops, edges forwards, stops a bit longer, pixelates (there's that word again), and sometimes continues.

Sometimes it doesn't continue, and you end up pushing various buttons on the remote and before you know it you are back at the beginning looking at the trailers. And then you have to find your place again through 'scene search', and it's never where you think it is and you end up watching five and a half minutes that you've just seen.

And people ask why Grumpy Old Men are grumpy. Why do they fucking think?

21 JULY

Big Brother. The world is reverberating to *Big Brother* on Channel 4. Well, when I say 'the world' what I mean is that the tabloids are getting themselves exercised about the latest bunch of idiots sad and stupid enough to want to humiliate themselves in public to fulfil Andy Warhol's famous prediction.

I detest *Big Brother* because I think it encourages people with the benefit of an education to make fun of the psychologically disturbed, and that doesn't seem to me to be a healthy thing.

However, part of the definition of success for Channel 4 and the makers of *Big Brother* is that people like me should be irritated by it. If we liked it, its core audience wouldn't. That would be the equivalent of listening to the Sex Pistols when you were younger and your dad saying 'What a nice melody'. It would immediately put you off.

For a long time I was missing the point about *Big Brother*, and then today my son Matt explained it to me. And now I think I get it.

It seems that the problem is that old gits like me think of it as a TV programme. One that you might potentially sit down and watch from the start to the end. In that unlikely event, people of my generation make the elementary mistake of expecting something to happen. We think that maybe some interesting characters might emerge, someone will say something worthwhile, maybe we might learn something, or maybe even be entertained in some way. There'll be some ups and downs, and eventually we'll reach some sort of end point.

These are some of the features old farts like me expect from a TV programme. But that's where we misunderstand. *Big Brother* isn't a TV programme.

'It's more like you are on your way home from the pub,' Matt explained, speaking slowly and in as simple terms as he could bring to mind, 'and you feel like dropping in on a load of mates to see what's happening. Quite often you do, and there's nothing happening. Maybe one or two of them are asleep. So you might hang out for a little while, then you'll go home. No big deal.'

So now I get it. I've got a few mates myself who are so half-mad that I occasionally drop in on them just for the entertainment of finding out what stupid thing they've done recently. Quite often they're not at home, have done nothing, or they aren't in the mood to chat, so I go away. The mistake I've obviously made is that it didn't occur to me to make this into a television series.

So it's all about expectations. We're old gits so we expect a beginning and an end, and usually something worthwhile to happen in between. The *Big Brother* audience doesn't care about that; they're just dropping in on a parallel universe. And do they care that it's the 21st-century version of bedlam – laughing at psychos? Apparently not.

24 JULY

OK, so it's Saturday and as I sit down at the end of the day I'm bloody exhausted. My wife asks me why and I say, rather peevishly I have to admit, 'Well, I've had a busy day.'

'What have you done?' She plainly doesn't regard this as a provocative question, but despite myself I'm suddenly feeling indignant. The idea – the very idea – that I've done nothing all day.

I was about to embark on a list of achievements when I realized that I couldn't actually think of anything. Yet I had, indeed, been busy all day.

After a while she forgot about this, but it continued to niggle a bit with me, so I decided to make the huge effort of piecing my day back together.

Try to remember everything you did today. You'd think it would be easy, wouldn't you? After all, it's just happened within the last few hours. You were there, for Christ's sake. Scary thing is, if it's anything more detailed than sitting on the sofa drinking a glass of wine and eating parsnip crisps from Waitrose, I'm snookered.

Anyway, I knew that when I started the day I was determined to clear out the garage. I hate clearing out the garage, but I also hate never being able to find anything in it, and I'm also slightly embarrassed every time I have to open it when a neighbour is walking by. All our neighbours are the kind of people that have their tools attached to the wall with a silhouette drawn around them. Little glass jars with nails and screws of various sizes. So I hate doing it, but I've sort of run out of excuses.

I went upstairs to put on some very old clothes. By that I mean clothes even older than the ones I usually wear. In the pocket of my old jeans I found a receipt for a portable telly I bought several weeks ago and have been looking for so I can claim back the VAT, so I went to the study to place it on the slopes of the mountain of stuff that's waiting for the day when I feel like going through my VAT returns.

At that moment I saw a parking fine that was going to double to £100 if I didn't pay it today, so I wrote a cheque for £50 and started ransacking the desk in search of an envelope. My stash of envelopes had run out, so I went to the kitchen where I found that my wife had made me a cup of tea half an hour ago but now it was cold. On the worktop next to the cup of old tea was a key for the office, which I knew I'll be looking for on Monday, so I decided to put it in my briefcase.

As I opened the case I spotted some batteries I bought yesterday because the ones in the remote control are all but dead. I went to find the remote control and couldn't open the battery compartment and went to get a knife to prize it open.

Just as my wife was saying 'Be careful with that,' the knife slipped and I gashed the back of my hand and had to run the cut under cold water and go to find a plaster.

Sorting out the remote control reminded me that we had a video from Blockbusters last night that needs to be returned today, so I put it next to the front door so I'll remember when I go out later. As I got to the front door, the post arrived and included a card addressed to my son that reminded me it's his birthday tomorrow. I went to look for my wife to ask if we'd bought anything for him, and she told me that she's bought a flashy pedal-scooter sort of contraption that he's been talking about for a month or so, but that it needed to be assembled. She went to find the box. It took me ten minutes and a broken finger to open the box because it was stuck down with those huge staples that never come out, and the box was wrecked in the process so we won't be able to take the device back if Matt doesn't like it.

Inside the box, alongside a large plastic bag full of nuts and bolts of various sizes, and metal and polythene washers, was a set of instructions. I struggled to make them out before realizing that they were in every language except English. I asked my wife to fetch my specs, which she couldn't find, so I had to put everything down and hunt through the house. Eventually I found them in the netty.

Even though I still couldn't read the instructions, I could now get a clear look at the diagrams that showed a list of parts, including one of those all important Allen keys for fastening the various bolts. No Allen key had come in the plastic bag, but no matter because I knew I had one that I had kept after the last ordeal by self-assembly we suffered at Christmas. I wasn't quite sure where it was, but I knew it was somewhere in the garage.

Which is fine, except I couldn't find anything in the garage. And anyway, I had to go down to Blockbusters to return the video. And get another one for tonight. Except that they didn't have anything I want to watch, so I got something with Meg Ryan in it for my wife to watch so that I could feel virtuous and get on with something useful. Except that I was too tired. So I sat on the settee and then my wife asked, 'Why, what have you done today?'

25 JULY

It's Matt's eighteenth birthday today. He seemed pleased with his scooter item; he scooted it round the kitchen a couple of times, causing deep scratches on the tiled floor and taking a lump out of the refrigerator door. My wife had also bought him some CDs that Lizzie said he wanted and a video game he's been going on about. So, naturally, we didn't see or hear from him all day, and this evening he went out with his mates.

'Where are you off to?' I'm thinking a pizza, the cinema, maybe someone's house, maybe bowling.

He looked at me as though I'd asked what language they speak in Italy.

'To get pissed,' he said, 'it's legal,' and closed the door.

27 JULY

Today we had what we refer to, rather satirically I always think, as an 'awayday' at the company. I say satirically because we were in an overpriced and totally crappy hotel about 2 miles from the office, but the consensus is that we have to get away from ringing phones and in amongst some flock wallpaper if we're to be able to do some seriously high-quality thinking.

It'll be a relief for all to know that I'm not going to relate any of the 30 or so things that irritated me during the 'thinking' (anyway, they're our trade secrets) because all of them were trumped by what happened at the end of the day when I came to pay the bill.

We'll leave aside that these people charge an average of £4 per person to provide a stainless steel pot full of hot water and a selection of poncey tea bags. Let's pass over the £20 a head that is supposed to cover 'sundries' such as a pad of paper, a pencil, some Fox's glacier mints, use of a lectern and whiteboard. Don't even blanch that local telephone calls back to the office are being charged at a rate slightly higher than that of a call to Los Angeles from a domestic phone.

No, my eye scarcely paused as it travelled down the seemingly endless list of additions and extras that had not made it on to the hotel's original list of charges. However, it did stop with a jolt when it reached the last item – after the VAT even – which said 'Charitable donation' at two per cent, which added another £15 to the total.

I called over the receptionist, an obnoxious-looking bastard, who probably wasn't called Dorothy but should have been because he appeared to have forgotten to remove the bathroom plunger from his arse when he got out of bed this morning.

'May I ask what this is?'

Immediately I can see that this is the mincing machine's favourite moment of the day. He goes straight into it.

'The hotel chain supports the Save the Children Fund and we add an optional voluntary donation of two per cent of the total to any invoice … ' Dorothy pauses, as if for effect, and then continues, 'However, it is of course a matter for your discretion and we'd be happy to remove the item from your bill if you wish.'

'So what that means is … ' I'm breathing deeply and trying hard to prevent myself from hyperventilating, 'not so much that the hotel chain is supporting Save the Children. It's more that you are seeking to embarrass your guests into supporting the charity.'

Dorothy is plainly puzzled. He pouts and preens for a little moment before knowing quite what to say.

'Well, I believe that the hotel does make a significant donation, but certainly if you'd like us to remove the donation I'd be happy to do so.'

'So what this amounts to is that if I am enough of a mean, miserly bastard to deny a few quid to some poor children when I can afford to spend all this money on being ripped off by your hotel, you are willing to remove the charge?'

By now he's got the measure of me. There's always one and I am he.

'As I say, sir, we'll be glad to remove the item from your bill altogether.'

'Yes, please do.' This dick-head is so oily that he leaves a visible trace of slime as he returns to the desk to adjust the bill.

I want to give to charity when, how and where I like. Not in public. Not because I'm embarrassed into it. And certainly not via a fucking hotel chain.

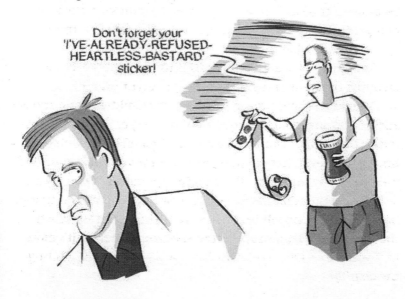

Don't forget your 'I'VE-ALREADY-REFUSED-HEARTLESS-BASTARD' sticker!

'The other one you get is pizza. You say, "I'd like the Venezia, please." And then there's 10 per cent on your bill for the Venice in Peril fund. But I just want a pizza. I'm not that bothered about whether the pigeons are destroying Venice or it's sinking in the lagoon or something. I just wanted the one with the raisins and the pine kernels, thanks very much. You know, I'm not really bothered about gondoliers, frankly. So no, I'll have the Naples, that's fine ... Have I got to save Naples now?'

JOHN STAPLETON

29 JULY

Britain is full of tourists from the Orient. Well, actually I guess it's fair to say that London is full of tourists from the Orient. Canterbury, Bath, Salisbury and Stratford are full of tourists from the Orient. Oxford, Cambridge, York and Edinburgh are full of tourists from the Orient, and most other places are more or less sane. Lucky them.

Over the decades we've seen them come and we've seen them go. A few years ago the place was rotten with hordes of Americans with huge bums, enormous checked shorts and even sometimes string ties and stetson hats. They'd whoop and holler about how cute the Coldstream Guards were and generally get up the noses of everyone except the taxi drivers, who got the chance to take them for a ride.

Then at last they all worked out that everyone else in the world hated them and decided to stay at home – by far the wisest thing to do, and we had a period where the only tourists, in London anyway, seemed to be European. And not many of them at that.

However, that's all changed again, and today London seems to be full of Chinese people. And Japanese people; maybe also Malaysian, Singaporean and Korean people. I know it's very non-PC to lump half of the population of the world together, especially when several of the nations mentioned have been in brutal and murderous conflict for several centuries, but let's be honest – to us they're all alike.

No, no, don't run away with the impression that this is racist, xenophobic, narrow-minded stuff. I know that all their language, history, cultures, etc. could scarcely be more different. What I mean is that in their incarnation as tourists in London they are all alike. In that they don't look where they are fucking going.

To test this proposition, try standing at the pedestrian crossing outside Buckingham Palace heading towards the Mall. On the opposite pavement, anxious to get across because the men with bearskin hats are coming, is what looks like half the population of Yokohama. Like the good and highly disciplined people they are, they're waiting for the little red man to turn green.

Eventually it does, and a tidal wave of humanity heads across the road towards you, apparently totally oblivious of your presence. They're not looking. They're not seeing. Most important of all, they're not taking any evasive action. Their ranks are not going to part to let you through.

So at the last minute you find yourself turning sideways, in that awkward movement you employ when a dog is going for your vitals, to try to narrow the obstacle you are creating against the anticipated onslaught. Actually, it now occurs to me that for quite a few of our Grumpy Old Men, turning sideways has the opposite effect, but that's by the by.

The same thing happens walking down the pavement. Regent Street, Oxford Street, Princes Street … anywhere with insufficient space and loads of tourists. A veritable phalanx of humanity surging towards you, making no apparent effort to break ranks to allow you to pass, so you end up weaving and meandering like a pinball as you try to go about your business. You might as well not exist. Bloody invisible. In your own city.

Well, sod 'em, that's what I say.

30 JULY

'Bluetooth at 10 metres.' Need I say more?

August

1 AUGUST

Imagine for a moment that you're burbling along in the car, there's very little traffic, very few people around, and up ahead you can see a zebra crossing.

There's a bloke walking along the pavement in the direction of the crossing, but he has his head down. It's not at all clear if he intends to use the crossing, but it looks as though he might.

You're asking yourself whether you are going to get there before he does. Probably not. Is he going to look up, see you and wait for a couple of seconds to let you go by? Probably not. He's reaching the kerb just as you are, and only at that point does it become obvious that he's intending to cross. Without pausing or even looking up. You screech to a halt to avoid turning him into marmalade. Even then he doesn't look around, but just goes on walking like you didn't exist.

Just how much would you pay to be able to pick your Kalashnikov from the passenger seat, lean out of the window and strafe him?

Fuckwits come in all sorts of shapes and sizes these days, don't they? Often they are fiddling with their mobile phone, probably sending a text to their mates, 'Wot about Arsenal then?' or 'How much for a hit of crack?' or whatever measure crack comes in. Presumably they're listening to the latest abomination by the Leprous Scrotes on their MP3. Quite often they've got a hood up; their New York hoodlum outfit. Maybe they are also on a BMX. Yes, that's it – hood, MP3 and BMX, three separate provocations that, when combined, ought in themselves to constitute a defence of justifiable homicide.

My guess is that these arseholes who saunter across the road in front of a Grumpy Old Man have no idea whatsoever of how close they are actually sailing. Just one careless flick on the accelerator and … Well, I guess we'd better not go there.

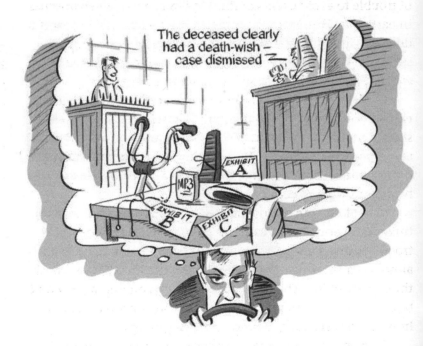

'If I stop at a zebra crossing, I stop and go like that [he waves] and I'd like them to go like that [he waves]. But if they don't, then I think, "Well, you bastard, this is the last time I'm gonna do this for you." I think we should be kind to each other. I'm happy to let them cross. I just want them to say thank you. That's all, and if they don't, well, they'd better be careful.'

DON WARRINGTON

2 AUGUST

Today we went to Bob and Carol's house for a barbecue. Students of Grumpy Old Men-dom know that we will go to an awful lot of trouble to avoid events of this kind in general, and barbecues in particular. However, students of having a reasonably peaceful domestic life will also know that very occasionally one has to succumb. If only to make enough of a nuisance of oneself to avoid being obliged to go again for a few months.

In this case, my wife seems to have more or less run out of excuses for why we couldn't attend. Apparently in recent weeks she's used up 'He's working', 'Mother is coming to stay', 'We're away that weekend' and 'He's got croup.' The only remaining option, she told me, was the truth: 'He's a miserable bastard and he doesn't want to come.'

I've told her on many occasions that she should indeed use this as our get-out. And with her closest friends she does. The trouble is that some of my wife's best friends seem to regard this almost as a challenge. Somewhere along the line they obviously think she's joking. That if I actually were to come along, it would be a bit of a coup, and I'd be full of amusing one-liners about how I hate everything. I'm not. I'm just grumpy.

Anyway, for some reason we can only speculate about, my wife eventually felt she had to accept one of these invitations, and today was the day.

Bob is an architect and Carol does a bit of charity work. Enough said? They live in a very small and very smart house in Barnes, which would sell for about £150,000 in Salford, but is apparently worth £1 million where it is. Which pisses me off before we start on anything else. The back garden is about the size of four double beds pushed together, but their designer has still found room for a water feature. 'Oh, how marvellous.'

There are already about 14 couples there when we arrive, so it isn't even possible to go outside and stand in the sun. Yes, that's another first this year; the weather is decent.

We are made a huge fuss of when we arrive, like anybody really cares, and I am given a Pimm's, which tastes awful. I quickly abandon it on a draining-board in favour of a bottle of beer. Carol is gushing around everywhere and eventually collars me to say that I must go and talk to Bob. I'm not sure why I must go and talk to Bob as Bob is a prat who feels more or less the same about me as I feel about him. If our wives were not friends, we'd happily cross the road to avoid talking to each other, and we both know it.

As it is, it seems that we're obliged to exchange some pleasantries.

Within three minutes we've exhausted all the fine detail of how his new gas-fuelled barbecue works, his personal recipe for barbecue sauce, and the splendid butcher in the High Street who always looks after him. Bob seems to be somehow attracted to the notion that he has struck up a rapport with a tradesman like the local butcher. I'm tempted to point out that the good relationship is more likely to be based on the fact that Bob has got more money than sense, but think I'd better leave it. After all, Carol and my wife are friends.

As soon as I reasonably can, I say, 'Think I'll grab another beer' because that's what men at barbecues do, and I head indoors. Spotting half a dozen people whom I don't want to talk to, I head off to find the bathroom. I hang around in there for as long as I can without causing alarm.

Here I must briefly digress to tell the story of Tony, who's married to my wife's friend Miren. Tony is the genuine article. He's so grumpy he makes me look like fucking Mary Poppins. Recently he went to a dinner party and got so bored with the conversation that he went to the bathroom and took a shower. Way to go, Tony.

Anyway, I usually draw the line just this side of performing my personal ablutions at parties, and after five minutes or so I feel obliged to emerge from the bathroom. Outside, apparently waiting for me, is Henry, who is, I believe, Emma's husband, and who drove me crazy when I was cornered at one of these events last Christmas. Henry seems to want to chat after he's been for his wazzle, so now I'm desperate to find somewhere else to get out of the way. The trouble is that there isn't anywhere.

Eventually I go and stand in the front garden for a little while, apparently preoccupied with the various standard roses. After 15 minutes or so my wife comes out and asks what I'm doing.

'Oh, nothing; just keeping out of the way.'

I can tell she's exasperated: 'But you're not supposed to be keeping out of the way. The idea of a party is to mix. Talk to people. Relax.'

This feels like telling Salman Rushdie to relax in the Notting Hill mosque, but I know I should make an effort and agree to do so.

Anyway, the next few hours are a blur of the new by-pass, the new Jaguar, and the new neighbours who are something important from Russia, apparently. There is an anxious moment when we get on to asylum seekers, but that happily coincides with the end of my fourth bottle of beer, so it's a narrow escape.

'Now that wasn't so bad, was it?' my wife says on the way home. I don't reply. 'Well, was it?'

7 AUGUST

Did I mention that Matt has gone off to Thailand? With three of his mates? My wife was, of course, near to hysterical before he left, and urged me to 'speak to him' about all the dangers that might lurk there. Since I was fully aware that most of the dangers she was thinking of are exactly the ones he was going in search of, I felt this was likely to be close to a futile exercise. And anyway, these days it's impossible to tell if anything you say to Matt goes in because he finds it impossible to communicate via anything more sophisticated than a monosyllable. Usually a single grunt, but occasionally as complex as 'Yup'.

Anyway, I won't go into detail, but in my own way I warned him against being persuaded in any circumstances to carry anything across any borders and to ensure that he was liberally supplied with condoms. After which I felt able to assure my wife that Matt was a sensible lad and had taken notice of my wise words of advice. Anyway, today we received a postcard featuring a picture of four near-naked Thai girls showing their arses on a beach with the words 'Fucking paradise' scrawled in Matt's handwriting on the back. Good thinking, Matt, that's calmed your mother down nicely.

9 AUGUST

On my way home this evening a car pulled up alongside me at the traffic lights and I swear that the entire vehicle was expanding and contracting in time with the explosion of synthesized bass guitar music that was emanating from it. Four black lads (are we allowed to mention that they were black? They could just as easily have been white, but in this case they weren't, so) – four black lads in a bright yellow Vauxhall Astra with the most preposterous spoiler on the back. Interesting word that – 'spoiler'. Like 'tin-opener', it precisely describes what it does.

No doubt the spoiler, which looked as though its last bearer was a Formula One racing car, was necessary to keep this particular vehicle from taking off – such is the extraordinary acceleration for which the Astra is well known. Anyway, for the moment the car was grounded and was alongside me at the lights.

Now I'll tell you the truth, which is that this stuff doesn't make me grumpy at all. Four black lads driving around in a mobile speaker doesn't irritate me even mildly. All it does is to give me a huge laugh. Indeed, one of the few things that consistently gives me a kick in a world where everything else seems designed specifically to get on my wick is when people go to so much trouble to look cool, think they have done so, and actually end up looking complete and utter plonkers.

What did these four guys think they looked like? They're sitting there, in a confined and sealed space, while noise equivalent to the second coming of Christ is going on around them, and remaining quite motionless and uninvolved as though nothing is happening. The noise is actually so loud that it's hurting the ears of people on the pavement, let alone in the car.

Because we're sitting at the traffic lights going on to Hammersmith Bridge, which take about an hour to change, and because I'm on my motorbike and capable of a fast getaway, I feel at liberty to take a good long look inside the car. It's fabulous. Leaving aside the pink leather trim and steering wheel apparently made out of a chromium chain, I swear to God that the hi-fi system must have been worth more than the entire car and all the occupants in it put together.

The speakers on the dashboard were the same size as those in my living room, and two more on the back shelf obscured the rear window altogether. I'm not kidding, this system could have rattled the spiders in their webs behind the cupboards in the most obscure corners of the Albert Hall. And what we've got is four guys – nothing particularly weird or offensive about them – sitting and not even tapping their feet. What, you have to wonder, goes through their heads – other than 500 decibels?

'One of these guys pulled up alongside me the other day, actually. Shaven head, tattoo round the neck saying "CUT HERE", playing this dreadful music; and I wound the window down and said, "Could you turn it up a bit, mate? I don't think they can hear you in Aberdeen." He didn't get the joke; obviously wasted on him.'

JOHN STAPLETON

10 AUGUST

My plan has backfired. Badly.

My wife came home today and said that she had booked our holiday. In November. Guess where? Blinking stinking Lanzarote. Why? Because the travel agent recommended it. A travel agent I didn't even meet, but who told my wife that she'd personally just come back from the resort in question and that it was 'lovely'.

I wanted to ask my wife if she asked whether the travel agent's trip might just have been free of charge, and that she was on an almighty commission to send as many unsuspecting dupes as she could. But I know that I am on very unsafe ground.

Serves me right, I suppose, but a high price to pay. One week of hell.

12 AUGUST

You'll never guess what happened to me this morning.

No, you won't, so probably I ought to say.

After riding a motorcycle on and off for about 36 years, for the first time ever someone knocked me off it.

No, it's all right, don't panic, I wasn't hurt. (Not that I imagine you'd care much anyway.) I was turning right into a side road, and a car was pulling out of the junction and ploughed right into the side of me. It knocked me sprawling across the road and into the path of an oncoming car, which fortunately managed to stop just in time to avoid running over me. Alarming for him probably, but not so alarming that he felt it necessary to get out to see if I was OK. No, for that to have happened I would have had to be fortunate enough to be nearly annihilated by a Samaritan, and we don't find too many of them in New Malden. A lot of Koreans, yes, but Samaritans, no.

Now I should add that these days I'm riding a BMW 1150 RT, which, for the uninitiated, is one of the biggest motorbikes on the road. I'm wearing a luminous yellow jacket that can be seen from outer space, the weather is clear and visibility perfect.

'So what was the matter?' was all I could bring myself to say as I finally managed to get to my feet. 'Aren't I fucking big enough?'

So I won't go into all this in great detail because it's very boring, but suffice it to say that the bloke was abject, decent, apparently genuinely concerned that I hadn't broken anything, and admitted total responsibility. Which is about as much as you can expect in such circumstances (and without which I would, of course, be giving his name and address in this volume).

However, it does shake you up, and it occurred to me only later that, in the absence of witnesses, it's perfectly open to him to change his story. However, we'll see.

13 AUGUST

Still feel a bit shaken up by yesterday's mishap, and find bruises here and there that I didn't feel yesterday. It's a long time since I've had to make a claim on the insurance, but by God, that's an industry that swings into motion when that happens, isn't it?

Maybe you've been through this more recently than I have, but it sure as hell was an eye-opener to me.

I reported the accident to my insurers, but assured them that the kind blind man driving the car was admitting responsibility and had agreed to pay for everything. I didn't need them to be involved – I was just letting them know because I supposed I should. In particular, I didn't want to lose my no-claims bonus, and – even more important – I didn't want to fill in loads of forms.

'Yes, that's fine sir. Let me just take down a few details.'

The idiot on the phone then embarked on a list of questions longer than there could possibly be in the final exam paper to qualify as a cardiovascular surgeon, none of which seem in any way relevant to what I wanted to report.

'What was the weather like?'

'Pardon?'

'What was the weather like? So we can get information about road conditions, that sort of thing.'

'Look, I'm reporting this as a formality. I don't need you to be involved. I don't want you to be involved. It's already inconvenient enough that some bastard has knocked me off my bike. I don't also want to answer a lot of questions.'

'Yes, I know that, but we have to fill this out as a formality. There'll be no problems, it'll just take a minute or two.'

Twenty minutes later we're still talking and I pretend someone has come to the door, leave the receiver lying on the desk and go to take a bath.

16 AUGUST

Today I woke up with a pain in the gonads. Yes, yes, I mean a real one rather than a metaphorical pain of the type I'm usually complaining of. It also feels a little bit swollen down there, a little bit tender and – how shall I put this? – a little bit misshapen.

So I did what I always do when something like this happens – I started mentally readjusting my mindset to deal with the prospect of imminent death.

Well, that's a bit of a drag, I say to myself. I had planned to start working a bit less hard this year and maybe take the odd longer weekend to try to acclimatize myself for the possibility of an early retirement. No point in going to the Boat Show after all; even though I couldn't come close to affording anything I'd actually want, there's now not even any point in dreaming about it. Pity I didn't get around to keeping chickens, or writing the world's greatest novel, or getting a record in the Top Ten – all those things I thought I might do when I was a bit younger.

I'll try not to mention to the wife just yet that she's going to be a relatively young (and also attractive and reasonably well-off) widow because I fear that she might start to think what a tempting prospect that might be, and begin looking forward to it. However, I know myself well enough to know that I won't be able to contain my self-pity for very long. I've managed to spoil my own day with all these thoughts of an extended illness and painful death, so I'm sure I'll eventually have to start trying to spoil hers.

This process kicks into gear at considerable speed and with remarkable ease. I've always been convinced that I was going to die before my time – and that's gone on for so long that I'm more or less at the stage where it's too late to die young.

Anyhow – let's be grown up about this and try to deal with it sensibly. I made a phone call and it seems that the earliest my GP can see me is Friday. That'll give me a few days to start 'putting my affairs in order'.

'I think that in youth you never view an ailment as possibly fatal. When you get an ailment in middle age, you are automatically planning your own funeral, and you wake up each morning in middle age with a profound sense of your own mortality, with the deck of

life tipping beneath you, the mattress about to roll you off into oblivion. It's a sort of queasy but not unpleasant sensation. And then you get up and it makes you nice to everybody for about two minutes.'

WILL SELF

17 AUGUST

This morning I had a letter from the insurance people thanking me for reporting the accident, and with five pages of questions, including 'What were the weather conditions?'

So I scrawl across the whole thing, 'I am not making a claim. I do not want to answer all these questions', and stuff it back in the same envelope they sent it to me in and put it in the post.

19 AUGUST

I take the BMW into the garage to estimate the cost of the damage. There is nothing wrong with the bike mechanically – I've been riding it every day since the accident and I rode it in for the estimate. However, there is a scuff or scratch on just about every panel, a broken mirror, broken panniers. Have a guess how much it's going to cost to repair.

Are you thinking £400? Maybe £600? Maybe you are unless you are a BMW owner, in which case you no doubt got it in one. Yes, that's right – £2300.

And, lest my life should otherwise seem dull, today I also received a letter from a firm of solicitors indicating that they have been appointed by my insurers to look after my and their interests in pursuing this claim from the accident. Would I fill out these five pages of forms indicating the time, date, place, make and model of all vehicles, had I been drinking and was I under the influence of medication or other drugs? Had the other driver been drinking, and did he appear to be under the influence of medication or drugs? Oh, and what was the weather like?

This time I called the number on the top of the form and explained to the person answering the phone that I don't want to fill in these forms. I'm not making a claim, and it's already inconvenient enough that I have to deal with the accident without all this bollocks.

'Yes, that's fine, sir. Will you just sign the form and return it for our records?'

I agreed to do so, hung up and put the form in the bin.

20 AUGUST

Another expression you never take any notice of when you are young is 'I never thought it would happen to me.' You usually hear it from people aged around 50, who are referring to the phenomenon that their parents got old, everyone around them got old, but somehow 'I didn't think it would happen to me.'

As a younger person, this sort of thing leaves you totally cold. 'Well, you should have asked me.' I can remember thinking when I heard my dad say it, 'I would have been able to tell you that you'd get old.' But now that I'm older, the expression suddenly has a meaning, a reality that leaves me feeling queasy.

Yeah, yeah, we're all used to the fact that we've started grunting when we sit down on or get up from a low chair. Yes, most of us have found ourselves exhaling loudly after a first sip of tea and having to stop ourselves from saying, 'Oooh, that's lovely.' Then there are those twinges, the various aches and pains, the stiffening back or creaking knee.

But there is one condition that falls outside all that gloop, and whenever I've heard anybody say it, I've inevitably thought, 'OK, that's the end, silly old sod, real old fella's ailment that is.'

It's a hernia. If you find yourself with a hernia, you've reached a genuine, no-getting-away-from it, pass-me-the-pistol-so-I-can-put-myself-and-everyone-around-me-out-of-our-misery moment. Might as well pull the blankets over your head and stay there till you expire, leaving only the smell of rotting flesh.

So that's what I've got, apparently. Not, after all, testicular cancer, in the cause of which I was busy preparing for an early death. It's a hernia.

As we've already discussed, I'm lucky to have a really excellent GP, who betrays not the slightest obvious sign of irritation as I go in with whatever latest piece of hypochondria has driven me to visit. This morning I assured him (not for the first time I might add) that I have testicular cancer. He gave me the quick once over and declared that I have a hernia.

'What's the cause of that then?' I ask, assuming that he's going to say 'It's an old git's ailment.'

'We don't know. Have you had a trauma in that area recently?'

'Well, I was knocked off my motorbike,' I recall. 'I didn't feel any ill effects at the time, but maybe … ' I'm hopeful. Being knocked off a motorbike sounds so much more glamorous a cause than 'You're a senile old fart.'

'Could be,' he says, looking unconvinced. I can see he's more persuaded by the old git explanation than any hell-raiser notion forming in my mind. 'Anyway, you'll need a small operation.'

So no imminent death, then, apparently. I am aware that I should be enjoying a bigger sense of relief than I am. It seems that I've got to go to see a surgeon at Kingston Hospital.

'How long will I have to wait for that?' I ask him.

He looks glum. 'Could be quite a while,' he replies.

'But I'm in pain and discomfort.'

'Yes, but unfortunately a hernia is not considered an urgent operation. It could be six months.'

Six months? I'm walking around with a bulge in my pants

that doesn't even have the virtue that I could disguise it as a very large willy, and I have to wait for six months?

'I'll have to go privately,' I venture. Being an old socialist and a child of the '60s I am, of course, against private medicine. However, my opposition to it is not as ferocious as my opposition to being forced to sit for 15 hours on hard chairs in long draughty corridors where the bottom half of the wall is painted in green gloss and the top half is painted cream, and every now and then someone has painted a Disney character on the wall.

He's not allowed to say it, but I can tell that my doctor thinks this is the wisest course of action. He takes a notepad and scribbles down a name and number.

'Call this and make an appointment. Mr Codpiece does surgery at the Old Albert Hospital on Tuesdays and Fridays. He can probably fit you in next week.'

27 AUGUST

Today is my appointment with Mr Codpiece about my little problem 'down there'. The one I have forbidden my wife to talk about. I have taken the elementary precaution of looking up Mr Codpiece on the Internet, and I'm not sure quite how I feel to discover that he has his own website. Mr Codpiece, it seems, is a keen amateur photographer, and his website is adorned with pictures he's taken of various scenes all over Britain. Actually, they're not bad, which for some reason I find vaguely reassuring. While scouring the site for information that will be useful in preparing me for going under the knife, I make a note of some of the pictures so I can compliment him with apparent sincerity.

I always make it a rule to stay on the right side of anyone who's going to prepare or serve my food, and also anyone who is going to perform any medical service for me. That involves a mix of some subtle creeping and a little bit of showing off about being a TV producer. The idea is to impress myself upon them as someone who is pleasant to deal with, but who would have no hesitation in suing and/or going public in the event of any mishap. Of course, I don't know if this is the effect I create – probably they just think of me as a pompous and pretentious git.

Anyhow, it seems I'm going to be in and out in a day, am going to experience a bit of pain, and have limited mobility and movement for up to about three weeks.

When I hear this it reminds me of the vasectomy I had nearly 16 years ago. On that occasion they also said I would experience 'discomfort' for a period of between ten days and three weeks. When, on Christmas Day, three months after the operation, I was still in so much pain that I presented myself at A&E, I was lucky enough to meet the doctor who had carried out the surgery. He seemed surprised to see me and unsurprised by the symptoms.

'But you said I would be in pain for up to three weeks, and it's been three months,' I nearly wept.

Do you know what he said? Honestly, I'm not making this up, these were his exact words.

'Well, you know, three weeks, three months, it was always going to be there or thereabouts.'

Three weeks, three months? Three weeks, three fucking months? I swear to God that was the closest I've come to chinning someone since I once got stuck in a lift with John McCririck. The fact that you get yourself ready to endure discomfort or even pain for up to three weeks, and then have to go through three months should, I would argue, count as justification for homicide. Especially when it's pain or discomfort about the area of the bollocks. Can we take a vote of the men in the audience? Show of hands? Yes, that seems unanimous. Thank you and goodnight.

Anyway, he schedules me for surgery within a week. No messing about when you're paying. Straight in. Yes, I feel a fraud and a hypocrite, but what are you gonna do?

September

1 SEPTEMBER

Another postcard from Matt today. Nice of him to keep in touch, I think, don't you? Loads of information, too. It was a photograph of a palm tree and the single word 'Blathered' written on the back.

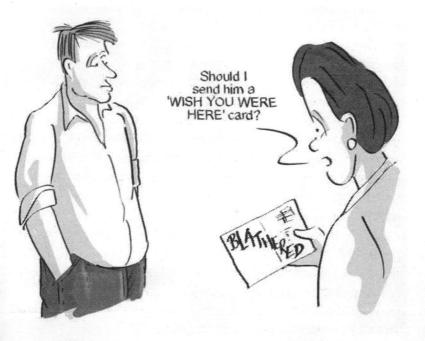

Should I send him a 'WISH YOU WERE HERE' card?

3 SEPTEMBER

Today is the day of my operation. I have had to eat nothing since 10 p.m. last night, and have drunk nothing since 8 a.m. this morning, so already I'm feeling like shit when I turn up at the hospital at noon.

A nurse, who seems to have come all the way from China just to look after me, shows me into a little room, which is rather like a hotel room, except with more handrails in the bathroom and fewer TV channels showing pornography. I'm handed a cotton gown that ties at the back and reveals a panoramic view of your bum to the astonished world as you walk along the corridor, and asked to fill in a lot of forms consenting to give my body to science in the event that things go wrong. (I don't think that's what they really say, but that's what it feels like.)

I'm given a razor and told to shave an area of pubic and other body hair about the diameter of a grapefruit in my groinal area. This is a new experience for me and I have to admit that I'm not at all happy about it. First, I'm not at all happy in any circumstances about a razor anywhere near my scrotum. Second I'm not at all happy about the pre-pubescent look this is likely to produce. Like anyone cares.

So, after careful consideration, I decide to shave the minimum area, just on the side of the operation. On emerging from the bathroom, the Chinese nurse requires an exhibition, and immediately declares that I have to remove hair from a far wider area.

'But I thought this was a small procedure,' I bleat, rather plaintively.

She smiles with something that looks suspiciously like pity and prods me back into the bathroom. After further shaving, I look curiously lop-sided like a before and after advertisement for hair remover. Except, of course, that no one would use someone with my body shape to advertise anything other than liposuction; but that's another story.

Anyway, I wait. And wait. Eventually I put on the telly and doze off. When I come round it's 3 p.m., I have a splitting headache caused by food deprivation, and I find Mr Codpiece staring at me with a benign smile.

'Good afternoon, Mr … ' He scans my file for my surname and I'm pathetically grateful that he gets it right. I'm expecting him to apologize for keeping me waiting, but he doesn't. 'So today we're doing a simple procedure to repair a hernia.' I love that word 'simple'. The more simple they make it sound, the more you worry. Conscientiously he goes through everything he's told me before, except this time he adds a couple of things.

'In two per cent of cases there can be damage to a local nerve and this could lead to a general numbness in a small confined area, which would gradually disappear in two to three months. And in another two per cent of cases there can be an infection, which can lead to problems, but nothing we can't sort out. Any questions?'

Now, whenever I hear anyone telling me that there's a two per cent chance of this particular piece of unpleasantness, or a one in a million chance of that horrible thing happening, I immediately know that this is going to happen to me. Do you? I don't know why they even bother to say 'It might happen' or 'It might not happen.' When I hear it, I know it's going to happen.

'So any numbness will go away, will it? Because I've already got my share of numbness in all sorts of places, and that's not particularly an area where I'd welcome a lot more.'

He doesn't know me well enough to know that this is my feeble attempt at a joke, and asks me where else I feel numb. He confirms that I am who I say I am, I was born when I said I was born, and then gets a piece of crayon and draws an arrow on the top of my right leg, pointing towards my groinal area on the right-hand side. Good idea, one thing we certainly don't want is an incision in the wrong place. No, that's something we really don't want.

Oddly enough, I have to admit that I quite like this next bit. If you are someone who more or less has to take responsibility for things for most of your waking life, the idea of being able to put yourself totally in the hands of someone else and completely check out for a few hours is rather wonderful. Especially for insomniacs.

I won't go into a lot of detail because you've had an operation, probably, and you know what it's like. I woke up feeling like the proverbial doggy's do-dos, with no idea how much time had passed. After an hour or so I was declared well enough to count among the walking wounded, and sent home with reams of paper listing innumerable dos and don'ts for the next four weeks. Most important among them is the painkillers. Must remember to take the painkillers, whether I need them or not.

5 SEPTEMBER

OK, so today I've been in agony for most of the day because I forgot to take the painkillers. Eventually I took one and it didn't work, and then I took another one, and now I feel like I'm experiencing the after-effects of a class A drug. Without having had the upside.

I spent most of the morning trying to pluck up enough courage to look at the area of the wound, and when I eventually did so, my worse fears were confirmed. The area is sticking out like someone has inserted a 38DD fake boob inside it, and my penis and scrotal area are all the colours of a Neapolitan ice-cream.

Fairly attractive sounding, I think you'll agree.

7 SEPTEMBER

So Matt came home from his holiday today, and guess what he's brought us back? No, I don't think you will. It's a girl. Yep, that's right. Apparently he met her at the airport, got chatting, she was coming to London but didn't know anyone and had nowhere to stay, so Matt said she could stay at our house. My wife learnt this ahead of me because she, against my advice, went to the airport to meet him off the plane. Matt broke this news to her in the arrivals hall, and she had to phone me at home to ask if it was OK.

Anyway, as I write this, Lulu (I know, I know, you think I'm making this up) is sitting in our kitchen drinking hot chocolate. She says she's 23 but looks about 14, that she has a place at a London language school, and intends to rent a flat in Earls Court tomorrow. Actually, I have a feeling that I know Lulu's intentions and occupation, but think it better not to mention it.

In the first exchange longer than three words for some time, Matt told me he thought he was 'in with a chance' and asked me if I thought it was OK for her to sleep in his bed.

'Yes, I expect so,' I said, leaving just long enough of a pause to ruin his day, 'when hell freezes over.' I made him sleep downstairs on the settee.

8 SEPTEMBER

When I heard Mr Codpiece say that I'd have to stay off work for a week, wouldn't be able to drive a car, and would have significant discomfort for a fortnight I thought what we all think in those circumstances. That's for wusses. I'll recover far more quickly than that.

So I'm not at all pleased to announce that it is five days since my operation and I'm walking around like C3PO. Is that the robotic one or the one on wheels? Anyway, the one that walks like it's got a broom up its arse. I'm totally knackered, watching a terrifying amount of daytime telly, and even falling asleep in the middle of Richard Madeley's questions. I could no more drive a car than compete in the Olympic triathlon, and must reluctantly accept that I'm mortal after all.

9 SEPTEMBER

So what happened to Lulu do you suppose? I see so little of Matt these days, and when I do he's usually got his head down, so I seldom know if he's depressed or not. Anyway, today he looked distinctly fed up.

'Anything wrong?' I enquired.

'Nah.'

'What happened to Lulu?'

'Dunno, she left.'

'Oh, didn't she tell you where you could contact her?'

'She didn't say nothing.' There was a pause and I knew there was something else, 'And she nicked my iPod.' I said nothing but had a quick limp around the house to check on other valuables.

10 SEPTEMBER

Actually, I'm not ill all that often, but this is the second time this year that I've found myself hanging around at home during the day, and it makes me reconsider what I have always thought of as the obvious attractiveness of early retirement. The truth is that I'm bored shitless.

You think you're going to get the chance to read all those great books you last read as a kid, or never got around to: *Anna Karenina*, *A la recherche du temps perdu*, *Bleak House*. What happens instead is that you read crappy Kay Scarpetta novels and fall asleep at frequent intervals.

When you wake up you make yourself an unwise sandwich, then you ponce about the house and get so bored that from time to time you turn on daytime telly. When you do, it's always two hare-brained presenters revisiting someone whose house or garden they made-over 18 months ago. Or it's a garrulous idiot helping a naive member of the public to auction off their family heirlooms for £15, which they intend to put towards the cost of visiting their daughter in Australia. Other times it's two teams buying a piece of rubbish from a second-hand dealer for £15 in the morning and having to sell it for £8 at a car-boot sale in the afternoon. And having to look excited about it.

At least this is only for a week. If it was permanent, I'd be obese and brain-dead.

13 SEPTEMBER

Thank God I'm sufficiently recovered to get back to work today. The wife says it's too soon and that all I'll do is extend my recovery period, but what does she know?

At the office I'm moving about gingerly. I was suitably evasive about my reasons for absence, but I'm sure everyone knows. No one acts surprised to see me. Actually, I think they all consider me to be so old that it's surprising I get about at all.

I'm determined to finish the day, but by lunchtime I'm aching and totally knackered. Although it pains me to admit that my wife is right, she is. I should have waited longer. Obviously, I won't be saying so.

16 SEPTEMBER

Today I'm more or less ambulatory, and I took my motorbike into the BMW dealers to have the damage repaired after recently having been knocked down by a blind car driver.

When I was first considering buying the bike, the salesman made great play of the fact that their service department would make available a courtesy bike when mine was brought in for repair. However, when I asked for the use of a courtesy bike on this occasion, it was explained that these were for people whose bikes were being serviced, not for accident repair.

'Why's that?' I enquire.

'Because we don't have enough courtesy bikes to go round,' he replies.

'Why's that?' I enquire.

'Because bike repairs often take longer than we estimate they're going to, so it's difficult to allocate courtesy bikes.'

'Well, if you made the repairs take the time you say they're going to take, that wouldn't be a problem.'

'Well, the trouble is, it always looks as though it's going to be straightforward, but then there's usually a problem.'

'Isn't that within your control?'

This is the sort of thing I find myself doing nowadays. Where once I would have shrugged my shoulders, maybe permitted myself an audible exhalation of breath, these days I want to make an issue of it. And even as I'm doing it, I know I am acting and sounding like a total fart. Nonetheless, I'm still saying to myself, 'No – why should I put up with it? Why should these people get away with all this shit?' And I can almost hear this poor bastard complaining to his mates at the tea-break: 'We had this pathetic old sod in here this morning … '

'So the meaning of the word "courtesy" as in "courtesy bike" is what?' I ask.

'Whaddya mean?'

Never mind.

The debate goes on for some while – I can't have the use of a courtesy bike, but I am promised that the repair will be finished to enable me to collect it tonight.

'I'll phone you at lunchtime to let you know how it's going,' says the bloke, and takes my mobile number.

By 4 p.m. I have received no phone call, so I call the garage.

'Hello, Tim speaking,' (like I care). 'How can we help?'

'You said you'd call me at lunchtime to let me know how my bike repair was progressing. Naturally enough you haven't, so I thought I'd ring to find out what time I can come and collect it.'

There is a long pause, lots of rustling of paper, the sound of murmuring and I know what's coming next.

'I'm afraid it won't be finished tonight. Can you collect it in the morning?'

'No, I need to collect it tonight as you promised and as we agreed. What's the problem?'

'We haven't got some of the parts.'

I remind him that several weeks ago the bike came into the garage for an estimate, and a full list of the parts needed was made and ordered. After a lot more going back and forth (I originally wrote to-ing and fro-ing, but I can't get the American spellchecker on my computer to recognize it), they reluctantly agree – like it's for them to decide – that I can collect the bike this evening. Their condition is that I agree to bring it back first thing in the morning for the final bits of the repair. I'll be in and out within an hour.

'Do you promise?'

'Yes, we promise.'

Yeah, right.

17 SEPTEMBER

So today there are 60 mph crosswinds, and rain is lashing down in biblical volumes (a vivid image, I think you'll agree – thousands of bibles falling to earth), but I've promised to get my bike back into the BMW garage by 8 a.m. so they can be finished and have me on my way by 9 a.m. It turns out that the missing parts are a small rubber kneepad and an even smaller BMW transfer, both of which could be fitted within three minutes, so I am optimistic.

The waiting-room for bikers is conveniently sited next to the waiting-room for car owners, so I am invited to wait in leatherette luxury while two pouting black girls, who look like part-time pole dancers, giggle and squiggle behind the reception desk and occasionally ask me if I'd like a cup of fabricated 'tea' out of a thin polystyrene cup. They don't express it in that way, but that's what it amounts to. Now I know what the overhead is spent on.

My personal theory is that if you are stupid enough to own a BMW motor car, you have already demonstrated that you've got more money than sense, so whatever happens to you thereafter counts as your just deserts. However, even I started feeling sorry for the very civilized-sounding French bloke with his wrist in plaster who had already been waiting for some time when I arrived.

First, one of the black strippers came over to him and asked if he was 'Mr Marseilles' (or whatever). He agreed that he was. 'Mr Reid will be down to see you in five minutes.'

'Thank you.' He sips a travesty of a cappuccino, winces, sits down and reads his newspaper.

Twenty minutes pass, and then the same Tina Turner look-alike came over and said, 'Mr Marseilles?' as though this was the first conversation. He agreed that he was.

'Mr Reid will be with you in five minutes.'

'Thank you.'

Already this bloke is doing a lot better than I'd be doing in his place. I'd have been unable to resist asking if this five minutes was the same five minutes it was going to be twenty minutes ago when she said he'd be with me in five minutes, or if this five minutes is another five minutes on top of the five minutes I was told he was going to be twenty minutes ago. And if so, does this mean another twenty minutes? Probably just as well it's him and not me.

Anyway, he doesn't do this, and another ten minutes pass, and a man in a suit that fitted him in 1995 and sporting a clipboard and wide smile approaches him.

'Your car is ready, sir.' Mr Marseilles looks pleased but also confused.

'Excellent. Are you Mr Reid?'

'No, were you expecting Mr Reid? I'll go and see if I can find him … ' He's halfway out the door again.

'No, no,' even the French patient's patience is beginning to be stretched, 'it's just that the lady over there said Mr Reid was coming to see me.'

'Well, I think Mr Reid may be busy … '

'No matter.' The Frenchman is close to panic. 'I don't want to see Mr Reid. I was just told that he was going to come to see me. Anyway, my car is ready?'

'Yes, just outside, sir.' The man puffs out his chest, further threatening the buttons on the already too-tight suit. Seems like some new year resolutions may be in order.

'And what was the problem?'

'The problem, sir?'

'Yes, I brought it in because the seat-warmer on the driver's side wouldn't turn off. What was the cause of the problem?'

The man with the clipboard looks at his clipboard. His brow furrows. 'Seat-warmers. Seat-warmers. No mention of that here. We've done the 10,000-mile service. Did you mention the seat-warmers when you brought the car in, sir?'

'Yes, that was the reason I brought the car in.' Now just a hint of vexation in the lilting Gallic tone. 'It wasn't really due for the service, but I said I'd have that done as I was here. Did someone fix the seat-warmer?'

Apparently there is nothing helpful on the clipboard. 'No, nothing here about seat-warmers. Would you like me to book the car in again, sir?'

'Can't you look at it now?'

'No, sorry, everybody's tied up now.' And yes, I've got a mental image of opening the door to the workshop and seeing all the mechanics bound and gagged. Which is what they deserve.

'Oh, OK,' says the hapless Frog. 'I'll take the car then. How much is it?'

Wait for it. Wait for it. The man with the clipboard is turning over pages and pages of stuff. And here's what he eventually says. Word for word.

'That'll be just £800.'

You heard right. Eight hundred pounds, and the problem you brought the car in for hasn't been fixed. And there's no reason to think it will be done next time you bring it in either. Plus, you've had the privilege of being jerked around for an hour or more. And, I swear it, several variations on this theme occurred just in the short time I was standing there.

And my bike? Well, it was ready after 57 minutes – just three minutes short of the deadline. An extra one hour on the price of labour, and to hell with all the inconvenience it meant for me.

Grumpy? I'll say I'm sodding grumpy. But can you wonder?

23 SEPTEMBER

Today I found myself in – would you believe it? – somewhere called Wagamamas. If you'd told me a week ago that I'd be prepared to eat in somewhere called Wagamamas, I'd have asked you if there had been a plague of locusts and this was the only place serving food for a 50-mile radius.

Anyway, I was out for a walk in Kingston with the missus and daughter and suddenly it was lunchtime. This in itself wouldn't normally have been enough to persuade me to go into a restaurant when I could otherwise go home, but I didn't want to mention to them that I was suffering from a griping pain in the general groinal area. I imagined that getting off my feet for a while might be a good idea. They were genuinely amazed, delighted and slightly suspicious that I seemed to be willing to indulge in what I suppose for many people is a fairly routine activity. My wife gave me a 'you'll need to explain this to me when we get home' look, which I ignored.

Anyway, having agreed against all precedent and better judgement to stop and eat, I had to steer a path around a variety of places I'd rather starve to death than eat in – you know the sort of thing: McDonalds, Casa, New Orleans, Old Orleans, TGI Fridays, La Bamba, Pizza Express, Est Est Est and so on. We had a narrow escape because Carluccio's was packed to capacity; I dunno what's wrong with me, but something in me rebels against being charged £18 for a not-very-exotic fungi. Anyway, the only place on which there was anything resembling a consensus – the least worst option – was Wagamamas.

Apparently it sells noodles.

It turned out that I was right in thinking this is slightly less of a hell-hole, or at least a different variety of hell-hole, than the pseudo-American burger bars that fester in every high street from Aberdeen to St Austell. However, that makes it only a relative judgement. It is still a hell-hole.

And – check this out – you have to sit on benches. Yes, that's right. Long seats of a kind that we used to call 'forms' when I was at school, with no back support. You then order from a scrap of torn paper something called Chicken Sita or Prawn Ramu (or maybe I'm getting confused with characters from Matt's early reading books), which come in a bowl and are guaranteed to slop generously down the front of the fawn cotton pullover I got last Christmas and am wearing on a shopping trip because I sure as hell am not going to wear it when anyone I know might see me.

All this would be bad enough, but at the table next to us they are having a child's party. There are balloons and cakes and streamers, all of which is kind of OK, except that the child's favourite present appears to be a drum. And it's not even one of those tin drums with the painted sides you had when you were a kid. No, this is some sort of ethnic number from the Africa shop or somewhere, which has a deep and penetrating boom that feels as though it's coming from somewhere near your spine. At first I was alarmed:

'Can you hear that or is it coming from inside my head?'

'Hear what?' my daughter replied. 'I can't hear anything.'

Now the other thing that should be said is that this restaurant, just like every other restaurant I ever go in these days, is already bedlam. People talking at the tops of their voices, waiters and waitresses shouting at each other, the kitchen sounding like someone has dropped a sackload of spanners down the up escalator and they're never going to reach the bottom; and all this reverberating around gloss-painted walls with sharp corners that do nothing to absorb the sound. In short, you can't hear yourself slurp.

'That dreadful booming noise.' I am now close to panic and look at my wife in desperate need of reassurance.

'It's the child's drum,' she jerks her head, rather more casually than I think is appropriate, towards the next table. I look to see the huge thing underneath the table, and the kid has one of those hammers of a type I last saw in the hands of that sweaty man banging a gong at the start of films, and is intermittently clobbering this thing with all the might it can muster.

'He's going to have to stop that,' I announce with a sense of urgency, and now both my wife and daughter are getting concerned that I'm about to embarrass them. 'I can just about stand the rest of it, but he's going to have to stop doing that.'

Now more suitably concerned, I can see that my wife is just contemplating whether she can explain courteously to the father that she is doing her care-in-the-community bit and is unfortunately accompanying a grumpy old bastard out to lunch, when an ice-cream the size of the Arctic Circle arrives and is plonked in front of the kid. This has the effect of distracting him for long enough that he forgets about sending messages by drumbeat from here to eternity. Crisis over, or at any rate postponed.

And here's the thing – not only is this place packed, but there are actually people queuing at the door for a table. It's drizzling outside, and ordinary people who don't look malnourished or suffering from insulin shortage, are queuing out the door to get into this shit-house. And remember (before the management reaches for m'learned friends), we've already established that this is far less of a shit-house than the other places we've steered past on the way here. Indeed, this is the restaurant equivalent of the Ritz-Carlton Hotel when compared to the other shit-houses we might have been eating in.

Is it me? I guess it must be.

25 SEPTEMBER

Someone has kindly written to me from Bedhampton to encourage me to add what he calls 'twitching' to my list of irritations. At first I thought this must be something to do with the wholly inoffensive and, indeed, to-be-encouraged pursuit of bird-watching, and as I start to read Mr Wintle's letter I'm ready to put him down as one of the many nutters who seem to think I'm the national repository of all things grumpy.

Usually they want me to share their grump about things like asylum seekers, whereas the truth is that asylum seekers don't really make me grumpy. The only thing I think about asylum seekers is that if they are seeking to live in an asylum, they sure as hell have come to the right place.

However, it turns out that Mr Wintle is irritated by something that for some years has been threatening to drive me to grind up someone's brains in a pestle and mortar, and is getting more and more vexing by the week. It's the habit among TV directors of studio or theatre shows of sweeping and zooming and cutting and wiping and panning across the action when all the audience wants to do is see what's bloody happening.

'Twitching' – that's rather a good name for it.

The most recent example that had me close to spontaneous combustion was *The Royal Variety Performance*. I forget the particular act – as a matter of fact, they were all instantly forgettable this year – but it involved about five people on the stage at once. Probably they were singing and dancing. Girls Aloud maybe? Anyway, some people you'd rather look at than hear.

Now by and large it's fair to say that I'd rather sit with my head in a bucket of hippo snot than watch anything like this, but for some reason we can only speculate on, now and then I find that I do.

It's obvious that the choreographer has designed the routine to be viewed from the front, where the live audience is, and you really need to see the whole thing if you are going to have any chance to appreciate it at any level. Instead of being allowed to do that, with the camera giving us the same point of view as that of the live audience, we have to put up with the TV equivalent of an aeronautics display, as cameras on cranes or wires or bloody trapezes swoop in from here, whoosh across from over there, tight shot, super-wide shot, fast zoom, tight shot legs, tight shot arse, until you genuinely feel seasick. And worse still, you haven't got the foggiest idea what's really going on.

Once or twice I've seen this happen when there's an act with a number of clowns or acrobats, where you can even hear the studio audience laughing or gasping at what they can see on stage, but you can't see it because the fat-head of a director is too busy showing off how clever he or she is to actually watch or listen to what they're shooting.

So why do they do it? Why can't directors sit there and do very little and let us see what we want to see? Mostly this is about showing off.

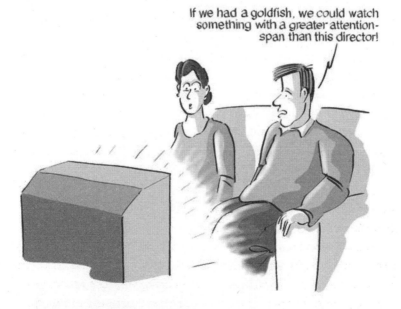

'It's as though people have seen too many pop videos and every director thinks, "We'll need to do 15 cuts per second, otherwise people will doze off or change channels." But *of course there used to be films like Papillon or Butch Cassidy, done with wit and wide shots, a certain pace to it that drew you in. Now it's all rushing about ... there's a gun over there, let's shoot some fucker there, he's on drugs ... you know.'*

ARTHUR SMITH

28 SEPTEMBER

So this evening I was ten minutes from the end of some dreadful film we'd got from Blockbusters when the VHS swallowed the tape. What's that like? You try to rewind and fast forward, and you just hear it snagging up further inside the machine. Now the tape won't eject, so you get a knife to prise it out. All this time your wife is pointing out that you're about to be electrocuted. Well, as a matter of fact, I'm not doing this for pleasure.

Eventually the VHS comes out, but the tape is still wound around the gubbins inside the machine. At this point you know that yet another VHS player is knackered. That's the technical term. Knackered beyond repair.

You're now doomed to have this happen about five times – ruining five of your favourite tapes – before eventually accepting that you have to go out and buy a new one. But it's not possible to buy a new VHS like the one you're replacing, and which you've only just learnt how to work, because it's old technology. New technology just means more complicated to operate, and more to go wrong. And anyway, it's scarcely even possible to buy a VHS player these days, but we've got so many old movies on VHS that I'm damned if I'm going to abandon them just yet. Except, of course, eventually I'll have to, and then have to buy my favourites again in DVD, and then soon that will go out of fashion ... How stupid are we all to fall for it? Like we had a choice.

October

2 OCTOBER

Can you get the lid off the marmalade jar? Those ones with the 'vacuum button' or whatever it's called. I nearly broke my bloody wrist trying to do it this morning, and I'm only 53. What's it going to be like when I'm 70?

Or the jar of baby beets? A huge top that you can't even get your hand round.

Worst of all are bottles of medicine, which you are probably taking only because you are in a weakened state anyway. You have to push them down hard until they click, then keep the pressure on while turning, which would be fine except that they still keep clicking round and round until all you want to do is smash the bloody thing against the draining-board.

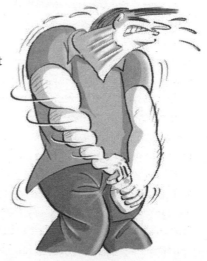

In the unlikely event that I do reach the age of 70, I'll probably end up being found starved to death, surrounded by containers of food that I can't open.

5 OCTOBER

I wonder why it is that after the age of 50, the way you feel is so precise a reflection of what you had to eat the day before.

Last night, bored witless by the telly and with no decent book on the go, I eventually resorted to a whole bag of hand-cooked crisps from Waitrose. Now this is something I never do these days because they are delicious. Even as you pop them into your mouth, you can taste the oil practically dripping down your chin. Nicely thick cut, some of them satisfyingly folded up.

But this is not an advertisement for hand-cooked crisps from Waitrose; it's a complaint. Because it is, in fact, a simple impossibility to eat one or two. They are the edible equivalent of crack cocaine. And like crack cocaine (I've heard), the second hit is much less satisfying than the first, but still you cannot stop.

The result is that the next time you look, you've lost your job, sold your house and are living on the streets …

No, no, what really happens is that the next time you look, the whole packet is gone. Within ten minutes you feel like you've drunk a bottle of corn oil – which you more or less have. Within an hour you feel you never want to eat another crisp in your life.

Anyway, that's what happened last night and today I can feel cooking oil coming out of the pores of my skin. And these days it doesn't just happen with crisps; it happens with anything.

Anything you eat that's unwise will live with you for at least 24 hours. Gone are the days when you could knock back 6 pints and a vindaloo and still go to work the following day – wretched, yes, but at least more or less alive. If I did that now, I'd be back in A&E. And now I come to think of it, last time I was in A&E that's exactly what most people looked as though they had done.

Anyway, if you're 45 and congratulating yourself that you can still eat and drink more or less what you like without much harm, all I can say is – enjoy.

8 OCTOBER

How stupid are you in your household? However stupid you are, I'll bet you're not as stupid as we are. Wanna bet? Well, how stupid do we have to be to pay extra for 'healthy option' baked beans with low salt, which just means the manufacturers have already saved money by adding less salt. Then when we put them on the plate, we add salt. Anybody else as stupid as that? No, I didn't think so. Can I get anybody else in the house to agree that this is stupid? Of course not.

9 OCTOBER

An advertisement on the telly this evening for something called 3. It features lots of little Pac-man type animations, and I know that it's something to do with mobile phones, but I have no idea what it is they are trying to sell.

This is a function of Grumpy Old Men-hood. The gradual realization that there are more and more aspects of the modern world that are passing you by. They're not meant for you, they're not addressed to you, and no one cares if you understand them.

This is because, as far as advertisers are concerned, you're finished. Written off. In the same demographic group as your parents. Ignore the fact that your parents are dead or in a nursing home, and that you probably have more disposable income than you've ever had in your life. As far as most advertisers are concerned, you're past it.

Why? It's not because the advertisers don't realize that you've got money to spend. It's because they reckon that you are now so set in your ways that you are more or less beyond their influence. Or, worse still, the thing you choose is more likely to be influenced by whether it's any good or not than whether it's 'cool'.

So you are unlikely to buy a Renault because it's 'shaking that ass' or a Peugeot because other cars are ashamed to be seen next to it. Unlikely to buy a Bacardi Breezer because it gives you the figure of a supermodel, or a DVD by Natalie Imbruglia because you fancy her.

When they started making advertisements for cars in which you didn't see the car, or hear anything about it, I remember wondering if the people making them had lost their minds. What sort of person would buy a VW Golf GTI because of a TV ad showing a fairly entertaining parody of *Singing in the Rain*? Or a French car because its rear end is supposed to be reminiscent of a bum? Shows how wrong I can be, huh?

No, in our day adverts were adverts. You knew where you were. I can tell how old you are by singing a few bars of an aria from Carmen, and if you join in with the words 'Esso sign means happy motoring' I know you must be over 50.

Remember 'You'll wonder where the yellow went when you brush your teeth with Pepsodent'? Now that's what I call a clear message. Or 'It beats as it sweeps as it cleans'? Another memorable line that precisely conveys what it was selling. 'Put a tiger in

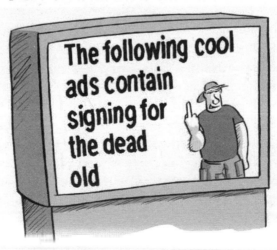

The following cool ads contain signing for the dead old

your tank.' Remember how we all tied little tiger tails to our petrol caps? That's what I call an advertising campaign.

I guess these days you couldn't make an advertisement inviting you to 'P p p p pick up a Penguin' because it would be politically incorrect to satirize stammerers.

11 OCTOBER

Another irritating feature of getting older is that any time someone says something, you start singing a song that has that line in it. Do you know what I mean?

I'll be driving across Salisbury Plain and the wife will comment on how rare it is to see a long stretch of empty road ahead, and I'll go into a few lines of 'The Long and Winding Road'. Worse still, she'll comment on the great gobbets of rain that are falling on the windscreen and I'll treat everyone to a rendering of 'Raindrops Keep Falling on My Head'. As we pass the river Avon, someone will point out the swans, and I'll give them three rousing choruses of 'Ride a White Swan' by T Rex. And so on.

The only consolation is that, being of similar ages, at least my wife and I can both sing the same sad old songs.

Even I am not stupid enough to speculate here on what might be the upsides of having a wife 30 years younger than oneself; but just think about the drawbacks. You'd be constantly making references to songs and bands and films she's never heard of, and thereby make yourself feel even more like an old git than you actually do. You'll refer to the Cuban Missile Crisis, and she'd look at you the way you looked at teachers who remembered the General Strike. Or you'll mention where you were when Kennedy was shot and she'll get him confused with Abraham Lincoln.

That's if she's studied history at all, which, if she's under 30, she probably hasn't.

No, no, my advice is to stick with a partner with whom you

have a shared cultural grammar. And if that wasn't my advice, I certainly wouldn't mention it.

12 OCTOBER

Today the suitcases came out in preparation for our holiday. Yes, it's only a month until we go away for a week, so my wife feels that we should start packing.

One of the things that distinguishes Grumpy Old Men from Grumpy Old Women is lists. My wife insists that the only reason I don't need a list is because she has one. Or, put another way, she needs a list because I don't keep one. Anyway, it adds up to the same thing.

The list sits on the bed alongside the open suitcase, and alongside both of those there is a gradual accumulation of things that may or may not have to go on holiday with us. There's a pile of about 20 T-shirts, from which at some point I'm going to be asked to select maybe ten. I know I'm going to choose all my oldest and most comfortable ones, and at the last minute my choices are going to be vetoed by my wife in favour of items without frayed edges or holes.

Less controversial will be the selection from among four pairs of swimming-shorts; only one of them still fits me.

In another pile we have things such as goggles and snorkels, suntan lotion and various medical preparations.

So just a month to make our selection, then.

13 OCTOBER

Bloke on the telly was attacked by a crocodile while swimming in a lake in South Africa. Had 137 stitches in his legs. 'Weren't you lucky?' was all they kept on saying. I always wonder about that, and always think that the lucky ones were those who stayed on the beach sunning themselves. Or the people who didn't go to South Africa at all, but stayed at home and won the national lottery. Attacked by a croc and 137 stitches – lucky? Not really.

15 OCTOBER

News this morning that the number of fixed penalty notices issued has multiplied by a factor of seven since 2001. The very next item in the London regional news was that the council is worried about the number of assaults on traffic wardens. Anyone see a connection between these two?

Of course, we've always hated traffic wardens. It's part of our heritage – a natural God-given right. But I have a feeling that when they first started blighting our streets, there was an element of their work that was deemed to be beneficial to the public. Perhaps this is a factor of the increasingly rose-tinted spectacles through which I view the past, but I think that maybe they used to ensure that people didn't park in places where it was genuinely inconveniencing others. Maybe they'd stop the traffic to allow someone out of the supermarket car park.

I also think that if you spotted one examining your car as you came out of the newsagent having popped in for a packet of Polos, you could holler and wave your keys. They'd give you a quick 'Tut tut' and wave you on your way.

Then, at a certain point, it all began to change. Maybe they were financially incentivized to seek out transgressions; maybe they were threatened with the sack if they failed to issue a certain number of fixed penalties in a day. But all of a sudden their presence on the streets changed. Suddenly, they weren't strolling along suggesting that you wouldn't be able to stay in this spot for more than a few minutes; suddenly they seemed to be skulking around corners waiting to pounce as soon as you were out of sight. Whereas once they seemed to be reaching for the ticket pad rather reluctantly, nowadays they seem to produce it and start punching in your details at the first possible second. And remonstrating, either gently or more violently, makes not the slightest bit of difference.

I saw an item on the news the other day about a bloke who was knocked off his motor scooter, broke his leg, and as he was being attended to at the side of the road by the ambulance men, a traffic warden put a ticket on his bike.

Recently I saw a traffic warden giving tickets to cars whose wheels were a couple of inches over the white line marking out the parking space. In the dark – a £50 fine, a couple of day's wages for a lot of people, for a moment of inattention that didn't hurt a fly.

So who do these bloody people think they are? And who do the people think they are who send them out on these oppressive patrols?

Eh?

'I had this wonderful thing in Ireland where I had my car – it still had an English number plate – and he came along and gave me a parking ticket. And I said, "Oh, no," and he said, "Ah, don't worry." He said, "You're English. It's a tradition. We don't pay yours and you don't pay ours." And I thought, "God, how nice is that?" But in London, you know, they're like armed guards.'

SIR GERRY ROBINSON

16 OCTOBER

I realize that I need to be a bit nicer about GMTV. I know quite a few of the people who work there and I really do think they do a great job. The only reason that they come in for some stick from grumpies like me is that they're on at the time of day when we are at our most irascible. By the time they come on air at 6 a.m. I've usually been wide awake for at least two hours, and up and about for one of them. I'm literally bristling for a reason to rant.

My wife and family have become used to this by now, and they usually steer a wide berth. Or do a lot of 'Yes, Dad' or 'Yes, dear' – but of course those people on the telly can't say 'Yes, dear' to me. No, on GMTV, in the week that Boscastle was swept away and some 20-odd cars were stuck overnight on a road in Scotland because of a huge mud-slide, the weather girl showed some movie of the rain falling in puddles on her way to work from south London.

I wonder if they ever imagine how it must feel to hear them recounting how they've had to scrape the frost off the wind-screen of their car this morning when you're living in a house where you can't see out of the windows for snowdrifts. When we lived in the north this used to drive us potty.

'A bit of a nip in the air this morning,' Eamonn would say to Penny or whomever, while where you live has 10 degrees of frost and outside you can hear the sound of people slamming their cars into lampposts.

Here's a tip, fellas. Not everyone lives in London.

19 OCTOBER

Had a letter this morning from my NatWest Relationship Team to inform me that they were moving into 'exciting new premises', just a short walk from their present location. Exciting new premises, eh? Well, we'll have to work hard to see if we can contain our excitement then, shan't we?

22 OCTOBER

I can make as many mistakes as the next grumpy, but usually I pride myself on not making the same one twice. However, that's exactly what I've done. I've made the same mistake for the second time this year. It's a big big mistake that I should have known better than to fall for.

When I asked my wife a few weeks ago what she'd like for a birthday present, she said, 'Nothing. No, really, don't get me anything. It's very nice of you, but honestly, it's just a waste of money. I don't even know what I want myself, so with the best will in the world, you don't have a chance of choosing anything I'd really like. So let's not waste money this year. It's silly. I'll get myself something nice if and when I see it. But don't rush around trying to get something for the day.'

So how does that sound to you? If that's not verbatim, it's bloody close. Would you have believed it? Be fair ... would you? Well, guess what? I did. I took her at her word, and didn't get her anything. Sure I got her a card and a box of chocolates, but not really a present.

Now you have to hand it to her; she's very good. At breakfast when I handed over the card and chocs, no casual observer would have detected for a second that there was a problem. There was no obvious air of expectation. No obvious disappointment. No empty silences. But boy did I make a mistake. It was unmistakable.

'Is there something the matter?'

'No, course not, why should there be?'

'It's just that you don't seem all that happy.'

'Well, why should I be happy?'

'Well, it's your birthday. I suppose that's why people say "Happy birthday".'

She looks at me in the way that I sometimes look at Matt

when he's being particularly dozy and I've run out of polite ways to let him know it.

'Yes, that's right,' she says eventually. 'It's my birthday. I'm 52. I'm ecstatic.'

Hmmm, seems like maybe a good time to keep my head down for a few days.

'The only time I slipped up badly I bought Mrs Stapleton a watch and she said, "That's lovely, darling." Then she said, "Almost as lovely as the one you bought me last Christmas." Moreover, I had not only bought her a watch, but it was almost the identical watch. Still, it's the thought that counts.'

JOHN STAPLETON

23 OCTOBER

Strange thing happened to me in Wimbledon High Street today. I came out of a shop and suddenly couldn't remember where I was. Wimbledon? Putney? Kingston? Richmond? Of course, even I got it after a few seconds, but it struck me that this is because every sodding place is exactly like every other sodding place. Same coffee shops, same building societies, same book-shops, same clothes shops, same electrical shops and same fast-food shops. And since every one of them is desperate to ram their vile corporate branding so far down your throat that it makes you gag, every street in Britain looks the same.

But it's much worse than that. Recently I was in Johannesburg – I won't bother to say why, because it's too boring, but the point is that I'd never been to the city before. I found myself in one of those McHotels – a worldwide chain that struck me as totally indistinguishable from many I've stayed at in Australia,

Japan and all over America. So I decided to pretend I didn't know where I was, to start walking and to look out for the first thing I saw that would tell me where in the world I was. This is a true story (not that anything else in this volume isn't true, you understand, but this one's important).

So I went out of the room, through the lobby, turned on to the pavement and started walking. Ordinary suburban streets, the sort you could see anywhere in the US, maybe North or South Carolina. Prosperous-looking white blokes, about an equal number of less prosperous-looking black blokes. Not much help. Street signs give no clue: Salisbury Road, Winchester Street. Well, it doesn't look much like Salisbury or Winchester, but let's stick with it.

I went into a shopping mall and there they were, most of our own high street banks, Starbucks, McDonalds, Burger King, KFC … I won't labour the point, but suffice it to say – and I swear this is true – I walked for 45 minutes, got back to the hotel, and hadn't seen a single thing that would have told me for sure which continent I was on, let alone which country or city.

So that's it then. The multinationals have taken over, and we're homogenized to the extent that Shanghai looks more and more like Houston, Wimbledon looks like Kingston, and every high street in the world looks the same. Well done, guys; you've cloned the world.

28 OCTOBER

Off on our holiday next week, and my wife says she 'can't wait'. When people say that I usually helpfully point out that they're going to have to. The holiday isn't starting until it's starting, so there is no choice but to wait. I guess you can work out why I'm so much fun to live with.

November

3 NOVEMBER

Waiting for my wife to be ready to go out this evening, I found myself flicking through – would you believe it – *Waitrose Food Illustrated*, which I hope and trust is a freebie. It was full of the usual crappy features designed to persuade you to spend 15 times what would be a sensible price for rice, and 35 times a fair price for olive oil, but my attention was drawn to an article headlined 'What to eat to help you sleep'. As someone whose middle years have been blighted by insomnia, I always take an interest in anything on the subject, so my eye floated over the very practical advice to eat dinner five hours before going to bed, with a tuna sandwich later on. Then finally, in a section called 'Professional tips for bedtime snacks', was the following serving suggestion: 'a fresh fig scented with a few drops of rosewater'. Honestly: I'm not joking. 'A fresh fig scented with a few drops of rosewater.' Go on, admit it, you've got those ingredients in your fridge right now, haven't you?

On which planet might this happen, do you suppose?

7 NOVEMBER

It's a funny thing about holidays, isn't it? Sort of a bit like Christmas, in that the idea is so much better than the reality.

This is probably a function of childhood, when the summers were longer and your idea of a good time was a day on the beach with a bucket and spade building sandcastles and waiting for the tide to come in and flood them. Except that your older brother would kick the sodding walls down just before the tide got there, ruining the work you'd done for hours and not leaving you enough time to rebuild before the next big wave. And your mum and dad would decline to intervene, no doubt sick to bloody death of you moaning and groaning about one thing or another, when they'd spent every last penny they had trying to ensure you had a good time.

The worst thing that happened on those holidays was when your mum scraped the sand from between your toes when she put your socks on, or made you spit on your hankie and used it to rub the residues of toffee-apples or candyfloss from around your mouth. Or maybe it was the goosepimples that erupted alarmingly all over your skin after the sun went down. Oh, happy days.

What is it now? Well, the worst thing about it for me is that I seem never to learn. How many times have I said, 'I'm never coming away again to a place I haven't been to before unless it's a recommendation from someone I know and trust, and whose ribs I can crack and barbecue in a caustic sauce when I get home if the recommendation turns out to be shit?' How many times have I said that? Eh?

This year I even asked a couple of people I know and trust, and got really good recommendations – one in Sardinia and one in Crete. But what did we do? We came to blinking stinking Lanzarote. Why? Because the travel agent recommended it.

Well, we're here. The Princess Yaiza 'Suite Hotel', whatever that is, at Playa Blanca and – not to put too fine a point on it – it is my idea of hell on earth.

Now it's fair to say that I'm never in a great mood by the time

I arrive anywhere abroad because I find the whole business of mass-travel so totally vexatious and soul-destroying from end to end. In our case, the flight was due to leave Gatwick at 7.20 a.m., which sounds like a reasonable sort of time. Then you start to work it backwards. These days take-off at 7.20 a.m. means check-in at 5.20 a.m. There's no reason why you should have to check in two hours ahead of your flight other than the airline people won't put on enough staff to deal with customers promptly, and anyway it suits the airports to have millions of people milling around for several hours before their flights with nothing to do except spend money on things they don't really want and/or to eat unwisely.

And who buys this stuff anyway? Is there anyone left in the world potty enough to buy a teddy bear from the Harrods airport shop for about 40 times what it could possibly be worth? I guess there must be. It wasn't so bad when there was any meaning to the words 'duty free', but post-European Union, even that has made airport shopping senseless.

Anyway, checking in at 5.20 a.m. means leaving the house at 4.20 a.m. Which means getting up at around 3.20 a.m., and that's if you've got every last detail of your packing and travel plans finalized the night before.

My wife, of course, does exactly that. Her holiday preparations begin about six weeks before the departure date, and that's if we're going for anything up to a week. A longer trip would require a commensurately longer lead-time. The suitcases have been out on the spare beds for the best part of the last month, and we have had to have the oft-repeated discussion about whether we should be buying some new luggage. Everyone except us seems to have very posh luggage, and ours looks like something her father brought back from North Africa when he and Monty had finished defeating the Hun.

'I think it's got character,' I venture.

'It's junk, and it's embarrassing junk,' she'll counter with alarming accuracy.

'Embarrassing for whom?'

'For me?'

'Embarrassing in front of whom – that we give a fuck about?'

She ponders for a minute. 'If we're going to continue to take crappy suitcases, we're going to have to stop staying at decent hotels.'

I know what she means. The supercilious bastards who insist on snatching your suitcases from you when you arrive at the other end, and then whisk them off somewhere, and hold them to ransom until you hand over a large tip.

'OK, OK, maybe next time.' I'm happy now. This debate has gone on for years.

In the interests of fair play for all, I should of course admit that what for many people would be the godforsaken hour of 3.20 a.m. is not especially a hardship to me because I am of course an insomniac. Indeed, I should probably also admit that I get some sort of unattractive pleasure out of being the life and soul of the party as my long-suffering wife, who is not a 'morning person', walks around like death warmed up. Particularly because this is so clearly a reversal of the usual situation.

It's also fair to say that the journey to Gatwick, leaving at 4.20 on a Sunday morning in November, was not the usual ordeal by jam that characterizes most trips to the airport.

No, the tribulations only began when we got there and parked the car next to the 'valet parking', which we had so carefully booked via the Internet. Eighty pounds for a week looking after your car seems a very good deal for them, but for us it's about the same price as a taxi there and back, and since the last time we hired a taxi to the airport the driver fell asleep at the wheel and damn nearly crashed the thing into the central reservation, it seemed like money well spent.

Anyway, we were just stopping outside the valet parking cabin at Gatwick, which seemed like an excellent idea, or would have been, except that when we got inside they didn't have a clue who we were.

I love it, don't you, when someone behind a counter runs their pen up and down a list of names, none of which is yours, just apparently to double-check that the word that's written down as 'Dawson' or 'Williamson' isn't in fact 'Prebble' after all. No, no, there are 15 names on the list – I can tell in a one-and-a-half-second glance that none of them is mine – indeed none even starts with the same letter, but this bloke has to run the end of his pen up and down the list, and all the while mouthing 'Primble, Primble', but there is no need for me to correct him because there is no Primble, Prebble or Passepartout for that matter. Not my name, and not anything like my name either.

'Well, I'm clearly not on your list,' I volunteer. 'Is there another valet parking company working from here?'

'No, no,' he says. 'You don't want Gatwick North, do you?'

Well, I'm fully aware that I'm going a bit potty these days, and omissions or oversights which at one time would have been impossible for me, now do seem to have found their way into my repertoire. However, even I'm not quite so senile yet as to mistake Gatwick North for Gatwick South. Am I?

I root around among the bundle of tickets, passports, currency, hotel vouchers, safety leaflets, insurance certificates and other general gubbins that threaten the necessity for an excess baggage allowance and finally find the 'confirmation voucher' that was emailed to me after I made the booking. And as I'm doing so, it occurs to me with a sinking feeling that inventing a valet parking scam would be a very good fraud, and I've been a total idiot and given my credit card details to someone who has cleaned out my account, closed down the site and is spending my hard-earned money in Las Vegas at this very moment.

'Gatwick Valet Parking,' I announce. And just at that moment I hear …

'Mr Preebie?' A stout women in a blue uniform is standing behind me with a clipboard. She looks and sounds like the woman who is going to be standing at the gates of hell when eventually I arrive there, flexing a piece of cane with electrified barbed wire wrapped around it. 'We've been expecting you.' Yep, that's exactly what she's going to say too.

With a loud sigh of relief, I hand her my keys and simultaneously think that it's an even better scam to take your credit card details off the Internet and then drive off with your car, never to be seen or heard of again. Can you imagine explaining that to the police?

'You did what, sir? Just handed over the keys to someone you'd never met because they said they were going to park it for you?'

'Well, I gave them money … '

Anyway, we'll soon know if my fears turn out to be justified. Meanwhile, of course, I don't have a £1 coin and can't rent one of those luggage trolleys with the squeaky wheels, so I have to drag my two suitcases, both with squeaky wheels, while my shoulder bag is digging into my shoulder giving me the gait of the hunchback of Notre Dame. It's now 5.10 a.m. and we're nice and early for the check-in, so at least we'll be able to get that over with and go and find some breakfast.

We consult the monitors. Lanzarote. Lanzarote. Yes, there it is, alongside 15 other destinations, all of which have been assigned a check-in desk except for ours, even though some of them are leaving as much as an hour later than we are. Against our flight it says WAIT IN LOUNGE.

We 'wait in lounge' with a few of the other early birds and gradually see the place filling up with couples, then families, then coach parties, then trainloads of people squinting at the board much as we did 40 minutes ago and declaring, 'There's no check-in desk for Lanzarote.' By now it's 6 a.m. and we are, of course, delighted that we've been up and out of bed for more than two and a half hours already and we haven't even reached the check-in desk yet.

Half an hour later, with about a million more people than can get on to a plane staring up at the monitors, they suddenly indicate 'Check in at desk 366' and the surge of humanity towards the indicated area resembles those shots of wildebeest that you so frequently see trying to cross the river. Such is the panic that the young, the old and the infirm are trampled underfoot with all the compassion of something with no compassion whatsoever. And yes, you've guessed it, by the time we get to check-in desk 366 there are about a thousand people ahead of us, and only one pale and languid-looking woman at the desk checking people in.

Meanwhile, of course, half a dozen smug-looking couples are queuing at the desk next door, which says 'Euro-traveller'. Well, after all, they've paid about twice what everyone else has for more or less the same trip, so they'd better get their kicks where they can. When the queue of show-offs has been dealt with, does the desk go over to helping with the thousands of plebeians? Does it bog roll.

Anyway, you've done it and we've done it, and eventually we get to the front of the queue.

'Did you pack your own suitcases?'

Now I know this is a time when you aren't allowed to joke. You just aren't. There is nothing funny about it, and even if you weren't going to be arrested and featured on the front page of the *Sun* for being a bloody idiot, there would be plenty of reasons to avoid any of the responses that she's heard so many times before. Ranging, no doubt, from 'No, of course my valet did the packing' to 'We have this bloke who comes in; wears a white sheet and a pink chequered flag on his head, dark glasses.'

So instead you put on your most responsible and grown-up voice and say yes.

'Did anyone give you anything to take with you?'

Your mind is saying, 'Well, just this little package tied up with cellophane and a battery and clock,' but that way lies madness, a long jail sentence and public ridicule. So you hear yourself say 'No'.

'Do you have any of these items in your hand luggage?'

You cast your eye down the list and ask yourself, 'Did I pack the carving knife or the machete?' but quickly answer 'No'.

'Window or aisle?'

We glance at each other and answer hopefully, 'One of each?'

'I've got no seats together now I'm afraid,' implying that it's our fault; we should have arrived here earlier. 'I can put one of you in row 13 and the other in row 28 if that's any good, but the plane is full today and that's the best I can do.'

So round about now you're ready to go off on one for the first of what will no doubt be many times in the coming week. On the other hand, you've seen so many of those programmes about easyJet, and marvelled how anyone can be so half-witted that they think the airline could give a toss that you are ranting and raving and making a prat of yourself, that you just sigh and nod. And anyway, my wife is probably secretly pleased that she's not going to have to put up with my moaning and complaining about insufficient legroom for three and a half hours.

'Oh, and by the way,' she says as she hands back your passports and boarding cards, 'I'm afraid there's been a problem with the inbound aircraft and we are experiencing delays. Watch the boards for further notice.'

'Any idea of the length of the delay?'

'Could be two hours.'

Yes, and it could be a week, but which is it? Yes, that's right, you think it but you don't say it. Two hours always means at least three before you leave the tarmac, so you could have stayed in bed till 6.30 a.m. and still have made the flight.

Most of the families going with you are by now making arrangements for the old man with the tattoos, earrings and skinhead holiday-haircut to go to the bar for a couple of pints of warm lager, while Mum and the kids go and eat burger and chips. Because we're snobs we decide to go to Hi Sushi and have something exotic, expensive and largely without nutritional value. We do end up eating far more raw fish than anyone in their right minds would eat at that time of the morning, and an hour and a half later we are mooching around the Harrods teddies feeling distinctly queasy.

At last the flight is called. You scurry off to the designated gate to find the same thousand people sitting in rows ahead of you, except that by now the old man is a bit pissed and the kids are getting even more cantankerous because they've been up half the night. The plane is boarding by rows, and there is the usual division of people who can't wait to get on the plane because they think this will confer some sort of advantage, and the others who are far too cool to queue and who ostentatiously sit reading the paper or staring into space until everyone else is up and they are the last.

Being six feet three inches tall is, of course, the perfect height for travelling in economy. If I sit bolt upright, as if in a deportment class, I can just about squeeze my legs into the space, but only by having them digging hard into the back of the seat in front of me. And of course my seat has got to remain 'with the tray stowed away and in the upright position' because that would obviously make a tremendous difference in the event that we crash into the side of a mountain. Yes folks, it's time to give ourselves over totally to being treated like halfwits, and for the next three and a half hours at least there is not a goddamn thing you can do about it.

Once on the plane, I'm always the one who's going to be sitting next to the first-time flyer or the sweaty Sumo wrestler, who seems to have come straight from a bout, or, maybe worst of all, the proud father of a two-year-old that's going to scream for the whole journey.

Now, I never actually speak to anyone on planes. My wife says that I send out unfriendly vibes to people, thereby discouraging them from opening a conversation. I'm not at all sure how I do it, but I admit that I just think of this as a neat trick. However, because 'Dad' sitting next to me is so used to people being charmed by little Tarquin's ability to gargle, it's possibly going to take a few tries before he realizes that he has sat next to fucking Darth Vader. When even he realizes that his feeble attempts to engage with me are plainly going nowhere, I can eventually get on with my book.

Despite the very best of intentions, it's difficult to read a book on a plane. I usually pack something I'm really looking forward to, and relish the idea of being in one of the very few environments left to us in which no phones can ring, I can't receive any urgent emails or texts, and I don't have to worry about moving the car because the meter has run out.

In reality, of course, you are crammed into a seat designed with enough legroom for Toulouse-Lautrec, there are kids screaming, and asinine announcements every few minutes repeated in three different languages.

However, you have to be impressed by the 'turn off mobiles and other electronic devices because they might interfere with the aircraft's electronics systems' trick. Congratulations to the genius who thought that one up.

When I first heard it, I remember thinking. Hmmm, this is a 150 ton goliath capable of carrying 350 people and their luggage

4000 miles, steered and controlled by the most advanced and complex navigation equipment known to man – far more sophisticated than that which took men to the moon and back – and we're supposed to believe that it can be confused to the extent that we will all plummet to our doom by a call from Maggie in accounts. Then I started to realize. Of course it isn't, but who's going to take the risk? And if you did take the risk, you can be sure that the other passengers would grass you up immediately for endangering their lives and that of all the little Tarquins.

I'll bet the train operators wished they'd thought of that sooner. And I wish they had too. 'Sorry, you can't use your mobile on the train because there's a risk that it might interfere with the train's navigation system.' Oh, you mean we might end up in Portsmouth instead of Port Talbot? Better put it away.

No, it's too late; that particular horse has bolted. But thank God we're all prepared to believe the plane crash fantasy. That's a good one.

So we can't allow the moment to pass without a few nasty words on the side about airline food, now can we? We should, but we just can't.

Why is it, do you think, that we're all willing to eat stuff on a plane that we wouldn't dream of eating back at home, even if we hadn't eaten since Michaelmas? What is that about? Is it because you've paid for it as part of the ticket price and so you think it's free? I hope not. Is it because it smells better than it tastes? Maybe partially. I'm stumped for an explanation, and as the trolley starts at the front end of the gangway, you find your-self thinking, 'No, no, I'm already feeling ill after that sodding sushi; there's no way on earth I'm going to eat that rubbish.' Then, as it gets closer, you think, well maybe I'll just have the fruit and the tea. Or maybe just that delicious white bread roll. Then they come up alongside you and you see the tin-foil container and the smell gets stronger and they say, 'Would you like some breakfast, sir?' and you hear yourself say, 'Yes'.

I always regret it. Every single time without fail I regret it. A lump of something yellow, the shape and consistency of a sheep's tongue, which they call an omelette, a round stick of processed and reprocessed crap, which they call a sausage, a half of something that was once a tomato, and a 'potato croquette'. All produced in their tens of thousand every day from the finest possible ingredients. Ugh. I'm at risk of throwing up just describing it. And yet …

The pilot comes on the speaker to warn us that there is a 'bit of turbulence' at our destination, but nothing to worry about. Everyone around me looks apprehensive, but I've been blessed with a disposition that never worries about dying in a plane crash. I always think that when the pilot comes on and says, 'Sorry folks, all the systems have failed and we haven't a prayer,' I'm just going to experience an enormous surge of relief that it's all about to be over and there is not a thing I can do about it.

Anyway, now we're coming in to land. I'm feeling bilious and the rapid descent is making my ears pop. Everyone is looking out of the windows and oohing and aahing like they've never seen the sea before. After wobbling about, tilting and correcting in what seem like gale-force winds outside, we come down on the tarmac with the kind of bang you'd expect to feel if we'd been dropped over a cliff. All the luggage lockers fly open, depositing various bits of debris on the heads of the passengers. There is a momentary sense of shared alarm from our near-death experience and then, wait for it, there is spontaneous applause. That's great, isn't it? 'Well done, we're alive and not sprawled all over the runway at a foreign airport with our smalls, intestines and beach towels blowing around our ears.' Let's applaud!

A surly-looking man with a cigarette waves us through passport control because we're all part of the European Community nowadays, and it's off to the conveyer belt to look out for the luggage. It doesn't matter if you checked in first, last or somewhere in the middle, your luggage is always going to come off the conveyer belt last or, as an occasional variation on the theme, one of your cases is going to come off early and the other one is going to come off late. And in between the two events you are going to be spending a happy 20 minutes speculating on how that could happen.

Why do men always want to get so close to the edge of the conveyor belt? This takes us into 'roasting meat at barbecues' and 'hogging the remote control' territory. There is something macho or 'alpha male' about it. It takes a supreme effort of will just to stand back and watch, and then step forward to snatch your case off the moving runway. Watch out for it next time. It's a weird one.

Anyway, somehow we overcome our embarrassment and admit that these cases, which look as though they were last used by Jules Verne, are ours, and we find a taxi to take us to our hotel. The driver thinks he's at Le Mans, and overtakes everything from donkeys burdened under what looks like five tonnes of twigs to trans-European coaches at 120 kpm. At one time I'd suffer this sort of thing in anxious silence, but these days I always intervene.

'We're not in any hurry,' I say, which of course makes no difference to him because he's in a hurry to get you to your destination, pick up an enormous tip because this is your first transaction and you didn't bring any small-denomination bills, and get back to the airport to collect the people still waiting for their art collection or windsurfer to come out of the hold.

Or maybe you are with loads of other people on a coach, which inevitably stops at their hotels on the way to your hotel, which is always the last one on the route. At each stop you peer out of the window at the rows of flags from all countries, and the uniformed guards running about to greet people getting off the coach. Sometimes you recognize a hotel from the brochure and think that maybe you should have stayed there after all, except that it was twice the price you paid.

Eventually, when everyone else has disembarked, the driver will look around and almost imperceptibly shrug his shoulders as if he's thinking, 'So these are the mugs who haven't heard that the Hotel Splendide isn't finished yet.'

Anyway, it turns out that our 'Hotel Splendide' is finished, more or less, isn't too bad, and if they can only remember to clean out the pool once in a while, it seems possible that we might have a good time.

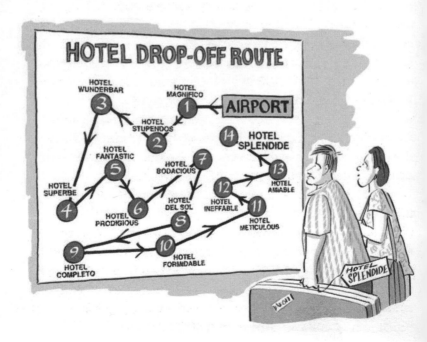

8 NOVEMBER

There is something uniquely unattractive, isn't there, about buffet-style breakfasts in these places? Even in fairly decent hotels, it's pretty damned well-nigh impossible to produce huge amounts of scrambled egg that remain recognizable for more than about ten minutes. If you produce a vast vat of it, and then turn it out in a tepid ambient temperature for half an hour, it looks and tastes like sludge. But that's not the half of it, is it?

Why is the bacon always cooked and served in bucketloads of grease, and why does it always end up in those curly shapes that we seem to have learnt from the Americans? And why is it always overcooked, undercooked, or cooked reasonably well but stone cold?

And what about sausages in any European hotel? They always seem to have been made out of chicken purée and be the colour and consistency of dogshit that has been bleached in the sun. Or they are those odd frankfurter-style things, which seem to be favoured only by Germans for dipping in their beer or by Americans for hotdogs.

The tomatoes are overcooked and have deteriorated into mush, the mushrooms are cold and oozing grease or 'brine', and the baked beans are barely warm and of a hue and texture that do not occur in nature.

And yet people eat it all anyway. And not only do they eat it, they swarm like a plague of locusts around the counters, as though they've just been let out of Auschwitz and this is the last meal before the world is to be plunged into a 20-year famine.

These situations do not bring out the best in people, and, in particular, they do not bring out the best in the British. What are we bloody like, eh? Have a look around and you can tell the British families in the hotel from half a mile away.

It's not just the pasty skin that looks as though it hasn't seen the sun since that day we tucked our trousers up above our knees in Scarborough a year last July. It's not the catastrophic choice of T-shirt with soft collar and loud stripes tucked into huge shorts from Marks & Spencer. It's not even the inevitable inappropriate socks and sandals. Sure it's all of those, but it's also the depressing combination of very short holiday haircut, tattoos on arms, hands, shoulders or legs, and earrings for men, which are supposed to say 'I know I look like a boring bastard, but actually I'm a bit of a rebel', and in reality just make you look like a fat ponce.

We're all overweight, we all look like oiks, and we've all got badly behaved kids.

Actually, we're pretty awful, but surprisingly we're not the worst when it comes to overfilling our plates at buffet counters. Sure, we'll have four sausages when you'd only have two at home, and a mountain of scrambled egg that'll keep you out of the netty for most of the week, but at least we won't then have a doughnut with it.

Lots of other nationalities are notably unendearing in this situation as well. The Germans are all fat, strident and not interested in queuing. The French wear their pullovers draped over their shoulders with the arms tied up in front of them and look superior. The Dutch eat ham and slimy cheese, and look quietly appalled at the manners and dress sense of the British. And anyone Oriental just looks totally bemused.

9 NOVEMBER

So the note in the little brown envelope in our room when we arrived said that we should meet our representative in the foyer at 9 a.m. this morning. Believe it or not, her name is Sharon. Having been on loads of holidays organized by tour companies over the years, I am a veteran of these occasions, and I know just what I want to do and what I don't want to do.

What I want to do is to try to find out whether there are any decent local restaurants and where you can hire a car that the wheels are likely to stay on. What I don't want to do is to participate in any organized activity of any kind. I don't want to be told about any local places of interest, I don't want to go on a camel ride or whatever is the local idea of taking the tourists for a ride, and most of all I don't want to see any local dancing in traditional headgear.

However, Sharon and her colleagues from over the years and over various continents always have other ideas. Whether it's because she won't really feel that you've properly enjoyed yourself if you don't see a lot of local manufactured colour, or whether it's simply because she has been financially incentivized, the Sharons are always going to be very keen for you to join in the fun.

Nowadays, of course, our kids would rather spend the week living in the cupboard under the stairs like Harry Potter than come on holiday with us – but when they did, these events always brought on family disputes. For them, the idea of anything from an evening of belly dancing to a Wild West rodeo sounded like heaven on earth. For me, of course, it was the biblical opposite.

Of course, even then I knew better than to refuse point blank to go on any of the trips at the meeting with Sharon. I'd try to get away with, 'Well, let's have a think about it. We're here for a fortnight so there's lots of time,' and then play it long, hoping that by the time they realized we hadn't been on any of these stupid jaunts, there wouldn't be enough days left to squeeze them in.

'Never mind,' I'd say. 'Maybe next time.'

Well, I reckon I probably got away with this once, or maybe twice at the most. All the rest of the times we'd have a little family domestic in which I'd be variously accused of being miserly or miserable, and I'd eventually fall back on something as pathetic as 'It's my holiday too' before grudgingly giving in.

Probably I should report that, once embarked upon, these trips turned out to be better than I had feared. Unfortunately, they were always exactly as bad as I had feared. Not better, not worse, just exactly as bad as I had feared. Always a rip-off and always patronizing to everyone concerned.

These days we're spared all that. The kids are at home wrecking the house and my wife knows far better than even to suggest any tours. So at 9 a.m. this morning we turned up in the foyer to see Sharon.

Well, it's a big foyer at the Princess Yaiza Hotel, and dotted around in the corners looking embarrassed are various pallid-skinned people, some of whom I recognize from the plane. They're obviously all waiting for Sharon too.

Eventually Sharon turns up and, if this were an interactive website instead of a book, you'd be able to describe her to me just exactly as accurately as I could describe her to you. Sharons come in only two different varieties. There's Sharon mark 1, who is young, ditzy, gushing, always rushing around, and gets her way with the locals by flirting. Sharon mark 1 is basically in the resort because she has a local boyfriend, or maybe loads of local boyfriends, and is to be seen sunbathing topless on the local beach at any and every opportunity. Sharon mark 2 could be mark 1's mother, and presumably was mark 1 a few years ago, and is now either married to a local man, or the old man has quit his job as an electrician in West Ham and they've been living out here for 'three years now'. 'Wouldn't go back. Wild horses wouldn't drag me. Mind, I miss my mates, and I miss Christmas, but other than that you can keep it.'

Anyway, it turns out that this Sharon is mark 2. Sharon has got a lot of little leaflets, a lot of organized trips to sell, and a lot too much foundation. We wait dutifully while everyone else books their adventures, after which Sharon can barely mask her disappointment that we are not doing anything she'd like us to do. However, she rallies when we say we want to hire a car because she can recommend a little place where she knows the owner and he'll look after us; and she's only too happy to recommend a couple of restaurants, at which we must be sure to mention that 'Sharon sent us'. I'm sure that's in order to ensure excellent service rather than to send any rake-off in the direction of Sharon.

10 NOVEMBER

So my main achievement today was to organize our hire car. I find it's as well not to have too high expectations on holiday.

When we returned to the room last night we found a little chocolate slowly melting on the pillow, and a message from Sharon saying that I was to meet the man with the hire car in reception at 8 a.m. That's a bit earlier than I'd wanted, but hey, I don't want to be the one to complain about anyone being too early. I arrive at reception at 8 a.m. and, to be fair, so does the bloke from the car hire company. I proffer my driving licence, but he is confused. No, no, he doesn't have my car with him, and I am to accompany him to the local office.

I've told my wife that I'll only be five minutes, but I'm too far from the room to go back and tell her I'll be longer, and anyway, how long can this take?

We go out into the car park and get into a rusty, once-white Seat with no hubcaps and speed off into the town, taking no apparent notice of road signs, pedestrians, stray dogs or children. I'm trying to pay attention because I have an idea that I'm going to have to drive this route in reverse, and wish I'd saved a couple of bread rolls from breakfast so I could have laid a trail of crumbs out of the window. After about 15 minutes I am totally lost.

Now we are hurtling down very narrow streets with washing

hanging out overhead and it reminds me of nothing more than a scene from *The Italian Job*. The original one – and that's another thing …

Eventually, we squeal to a halt in what passes for a car park and my escort gestures towards a little door into a building with no signs outside and no windows. Inside I find half a dozen couples of various nationalities distributed around the office in no particular order, while a fat sweaty man in a T-shirt, who looks like an extra from *Casablanca* and is only short of the fez, bellows down the telephone in Spanish. This goes on for five minutes or so, during which several of the couples exchange looks, and eventually our host slams down the receiver, looks up, decides who is first, and then speaks to them in apparently perfectly fluent German. They reply. There is a brief exchange. In German. It appears that he has not got what they want and have been led to expect, so with lots of loud exhaling and more of those looks, they walk out and slam the door. He looks at us as if in appeal, and we respond by tut-tutting as though whatever is the problem, it must be the fault of the Germans. We all know what they're like.

The next couple appear to be French, and now I'm rather impressed that he begins to address them at great speed and volume in what is apparently fluent French. However, this time he is only two sentences into the conversation when the phone rings again; he picks it up and, without pause, starts bellowing into it again in Spanish. This goes on for a while, during which everyone in the shop is getting fed up. Including me, but since I have no obvious way of getting back to the hotel, I decide to stick it out. Maybe an hour has passed since I said I'd be gone for five minutes. This may be, after all, what is meant by the 'local colour' that my wife is always telling me we should see more of.

Eventually, the French people are dealt with, then the Dutch, then more Germans, and finally it's my turn.

'Ah, you are with Sharon,' he declares warmly and in very good English. 'You should have said. I have your car ready.'

A flunkey takes me back to the car park and I'm led to the smallest vehicle I've ever been in – including the Heinkel bubble car I had when I was a student. However, rather than remonstrate or make any fuss at this point, it'll suit my current purpose, which is to get the hell out of here as fast as possible.

I quickly master the three controls on the car – forward, back and brake – and navigate a maze of tiny lanes and unmade roads, and eventually get back to the coast, and from here I can get back to the hotel. It's now an hour and 45 minutes since I said I'd be gone for five, and am fully expecting anxiety, maybe a search party, certainly a list of worried questions. Instead, she hardly glances up:

'You've been a long time.'

At this point my wife says that it's too hot to be driving, so maybe we should take a walk today and explore the island tomorrow.

11 NOVEMBER

We did, and in the unlikely event that you are thinking of going, allow me to assist you in your decision. Playa Blanca is a building site. Playa Blanca is a vast, sprawling retirement community that seems to be designed more or less solely for the British. Don't go there. It isn't finished, and even when it is finished, it will still be a dump.

12 NOVEMBER

Now you'd think, wouldn't you, that having enjoyed the experience of the car hire company as recommended by Sharon, we'd avoid her recommendation for dinner at all costs. Not us.

We're so feeble that we don't want to run into Sharon later in the holiday and admit that we were terrified to try out her suggestion. So we go to Pedro's. Yes, yes, I know that sounds very unlikely, but trust me. The name of the restaurant was Pedro's, and it's on the sea front.

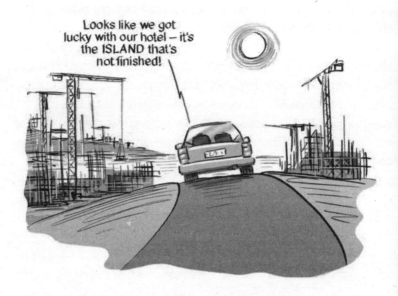

Looks like we got lucky with our hotel – it's the ISLAND that's not finished!

Every shop along the sea front is a restaurant or a gift shop, and this one is next to something with a parrot in the name, and you'd know it because – guess what? – there are two parrots chained by manacles to a perch so they cannot escape from the idiots and children who torment them from dawn unto midnight.

One good piece of advice that my mother gave me was 'Never eat in a restaurant where the menu has pictures.' I can't say that I've always followed it, but whenever I haven't I've always regretted it. This should have been enough of a warning about Pedro's. Pedro's menu is printed in several European languages and, in case you can't decipher what 'weal escaloppe' is, there is what I believe is called an 'artist's impression' of a large plate of what looks like spaghetti with a flat thing covered apparently in breadcrumbs and awash with a lurid red sauce.

Other delicacies include Pedro's beefburger, Pedro's fried chicken, and Pedro's 'all day breakfast'.

Whenever I'm next to the sea I have a weakness for eating fish because there is something in me that wants to believe that the fish I'm going to eat has something to do with the sea next to me. Maybe it came from there recently. However, in this case, the picture of 'Pedro's special catch of the day' is not promising. Not least because the 'catch of the day' seems to be a very regular-shaped item, also apparently coated in breadcrumbs.

Needless to say, a bottle of wine took the worst of the taste away. It was terrible. Don't go there.

13 NOVEMBER

Anyway, the main reason that we chose Lanzarote for our holiday is because it was the nearest place we could come to at this time of year and be more or less guaranteed some sunshine. That's what they said in the travel agent anyway. Needless to say, it's been windy and raining for most of the last three days.

Actually, in fairness, most mornings have dawned chilly but bright. Promising enough for us to believe it is worth going down to the poolside as soon as the bloke who dispenses the towels comes on duty, and bagging a couple of sun-loungers.

In matters of lounging by the pool, as in so many others, I'm always ready and anxious to start long before my wife, so it's my job to go and choose where we're going to sit. In making this decision, there is, of course, much to be taken into account.

The far side of the pool, for example, gets the sun first thing in the morning, but at about three o'clock it disappears behind block A, and is plunged into shade. And by that time all the other seats are taken. We discovered that to our cost on the third day of our holiday, but it didn't matter too much then because by that time it was drizzling.

On the other hand, if you sit on the near side, you're lying with your back to the pool all morning and, worse still, along-side the main path to and from breakfast. Not a good idea.

There are a few places facing the pool with your back to the sea, but there is a waterfall between the two pools, which even in a light breeze blows freezing cold water over you at unexpected moments, and you have to exercise maximum restraint not to yell expletives. The fourth side is where the kids' play area is, and is therefore out of the question.

However, the one thing I can rely on in a fast-changing world is that wherever I choose, I should have chosen some-where else.

'Wouldn't we be better off under those trees?' asks the wife. And now she comes to point it out, I can see she's obviously right, but something in me won't concede it. Anyway, it scarcely matters because after half an hour the sun goes behind a little cloud that's scooting at an alarming speed across what was until recently a clear blue sky. You grab a towel and shiver.

Not far behind that cloud you see a collection of clouds of similar size, and you try to judge the wind speed and direction to see if you're shortly going to have a few minutes of sunshine. But what happens is that as it comes towards you, that very promising-looking gap in the clouds closes up, and you are left waiting for the next one to do the same.

Joyful, eh?

We have tended to spend the morning by the pool, under a towel, reading our books while we wait for the sun to come out, and our afternoons driving around the island 'seeing the sights'. Except that there aren't any.

15 NOVEMBER

Got home yesterday. Nothing much to report about the journey except that it was long, boring, uncomfortable and I failed to resist the in-flight garbage that they call food.

I'm too old to worry about things like a suntan, but usually you hope to return from your holidays looking better than you did when you left home, don't you? Well, I don't. If anything, I look slightly pink, like I'm recovering from having just run up a flight of stairs. I've put on half a stone as a consequence of their delicious breakfasts. So all in all the whole experience has been just another reinforcement of my general attitude towards holidays. A waste of bloody time.

The only good news is that there seems to be a problem between Lizzie and her boyfriend. She didn't look happy to see us, which was not a surprise, and later it began to emerge that something else was going on. As I write, she is upstairs talking to my wife, and a couple of times I've passed the closed door and heard the back ends of lines like 'They're all the bloody same.'

Sounds promising.

17 NOVEMBER

Yes! Result! She's dumped Vaguer, or Vader, or whatever his name was, and thank God I don't now need to find out. I suspect I may not have been told the whole truth, but it seems he developed an attachment for Lizzie's friend Beth. The result is that Vaguer is history and Lizzie and Beth aren't speaking, though Lizzie doesn't really blame Beth, but she could have made it more clear … Anyway, none of that matters. It seems that Lizzie has given up men for good; none of us is worth a candle apparently; she's just going to get on with her life without any of us. I try to cheer her up by telling her that of all her various boyfriends, he was the very worst. No redeeming features. She agrees; he's going back to Ruritania or Kleptomania or wherever it is he came from. My prayers are answered.

19 NOVEMBER

One of the things that always happens when you go on holiday is that everything in your house breaks down. In days gone by there would be the odd crack in a window pane, a lot of apparently inexplicable stains on carpets, more than the average number of broken cups and glasses. Just to add a bit of variety, we came home this week to find that the boiler isn't functioning.

It's always one of life's joys, I find, to locate and obtain the services of an honest tradesman. We won't go into the whole gamut of calling them up, them being too busy, the egregious call-out charges, the sucking of gums and shaking of heads; we won't repeat it because we all know it so well. What I find most vexing is the extent to which you have to prostrate yourself if and when they ever do deign to come out. Loads of variations of 'Very good of you to come', 'Thanks for finding the time', 'I know you must be very busy', etc., etc.

My wife seems to have managed to persuade Mr Plunger to sort out the boiler. Mr Plunger is a nice enough bloke, but he's one of these guys who has to tell you what he thinks is wrong. And what the thing he thinks is broken does. Last time he came out it was the electric motor, which even I understand. This time he says it's something to do with the 'coil', which I always thought was a method of contraception.

Anyway, here's what all this is driving at: in my effort to make him welcome, I ask him if he'd like a cup of something.

It seems that he doesn't mind if he does.

'Tea or coffee?'

'Either is fine.'

'I can make both, which do you want?'

Then the bit that gets up my nose. 'Whichever's easier.'

Now I think we can do mankind a service once and for all here. We can make it perfectly clear that *making a cup of tea with a teabag is as easy as making a cup of instant coffee.*

There. It's out. One is just as easy as the other.

So guess what happens next. I say:

'I'll make tea, then.'

And he says, 'Great, but if you're making coffee as well, I'll have a cup of coffee.'

23 NOVEMBER

I wonder what they call a Swiss army knife in Switzerland. An 'army knife'? No reason. I was just wondering.

25 NOVEMBER

Worst day of the year so far. I came home early today, shouted, 'Hi, I'm home,' walked into the living room to find my daughter lying horizontal on the settee with a bloke on top of her. Which would be bad enough, but worse, far worse, it was none other than Vaguer or whatever he's called.

At the sight of me, both sprang up, rearranging their clothes – the only redeeming feature of this otherwise unremitting disaster is that they were dressed. Usually Lizzie's instinct would be to approach such a situation with aggression, but on this occasion she seemed genuinely embarrassed.

'Oh Dad, I didn't expect you.'

'Apparently,' I said. All too predictable, I know, but what do you want, a sonnet?

Later I learned via my wife that Varder (I'm now assured

that that's his name) had been so distraught that he had threatened suicide, so Lizzie had agreed to take him back.

'And the problem with him committing suicide was what?' I enquired.

Needless to say, I'm distraught. Horrified. And totally powerless. And best of all, Lizzie now knows that I think he's the worst boyfriend she's ever had, and she's taken him back anyway. When will I learn?

December

1 DECEMBER

Put on a pair of jeans today straight out of the wash and could hardly fasten the buttons. Of course, it always happens that your jeans shrink a bit in the wash and the first few hours are a bit uncomfortable.

However, I put on a shirt that has to tuck into my jeans and happened to catch my profile in the mirror as I go by. Am utterly horrified. The long, lanky bloke I've been for most of my life has left town never to return, and has been replaced by this bulky shambles, who's plainly too gross to fit into his trousers. I'm told that this phenomenon is called – rather cruelly, if I may say – the 'muffin look', which is a perfect expression because it accurately describes both the cause and the effect of the problem.

Anyway, the shirt has to go back on the hanger because today I obviously need to wear one that hangs outside the waistband.

At university I weighed about 11½ stone, and I guess I've put on about a stone per decade since. Being taller than average, I partially delude myself that I can 'carry it off', but there's no getting away from the overall effect. I'm overweight. I was going to write 'pudgy', but even in a diary as secret as this, I can't bring myself to embrace a word such as that.

This phenomenon doesn't appear to affect all Grumpy Old Men. Since the downside of excess made him give up beer, I've

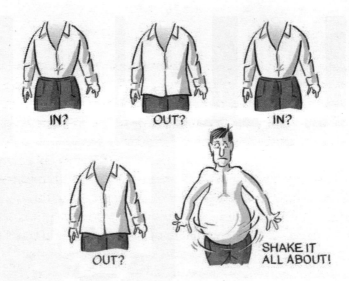

IN? OUT? IN?

OUT? SHAKE IT ALL ABOUT!

noticed that Arthur Smith looks like a fucking whippet. He's one of the few of us who actually looks fitter and better now than he did ten years ago. I'm very fond of John O'Farrell and Tony Hawks, but both irritate me by looking skinny and fit. Will Self – bastard – is skinny as a butcher's biro, but then he's still smoking.

No, I'm much more comfortable with GOMs like Rory McGrath and Rick Wakeman. Both with the same problem I've got; if we eat and drink what we like, we end up looking like rhino smugglers. So we have to watch it, which is boring.

Anyway, the point is that as the day wore on, the jeans didn't feel any looser and I realized it's that time of year again. It's dark in the mornings, the weather is wet and cold, and all the natural instincts are telling you to take on fuel to see you through the winter. Comfort eating to 'warm you up', which you feel you can do because we've said goodbye to T-shirts and are back into chunky sweaters for the winter.

And hell, Christmas is coming. We're bound to pig out when that comes around. Will have to go on a diet in the new year, though

4 DECEMBER

Well, once again Christmas is in full swing. It has been since October in most shops, but only now is the true and total idiocy fully under way. There are several home-owners on the Kingston bypass that compete for the coveted title of 'Squid-brain of the Year' by decking their houses out like a more festive and over-the-top version of Piccadilly Circus and Times Square rolled into one. These guys are using enough light bulbs to confuse airline pilots or to show up on the pictures from weather satellites. You can almost hear the humming surge on the national grid as you drive by. Actually, I think it's a danger to motorists, and that the perpetrators should be locked up indoors under one of the government's anti-social behaviour orders, with no appeal or parole, and no sight of the charge or the evidence against them. That'll show the buggers.

6 DECEMBER

Received a postcard today from the Piss-Pots Gymnasium advising me that my membership is about to expire and offering me the chance to renew at the 'discounted rate' of £50 a month. As I've been paying £40 a month for the last 12 months and have never been, I'm tempted to ask for a refund. Instead, I tear the postcard into pieces no bigger than a postage stamp and flush them down the lavatory.

7 DECEMBER

It's a week from my birthday, and readers who are finishing this book in the same year as they started it, might remember that part of the object of this exercise was to see if grumpiness eases with age.

The core group of Grumpy Old Men, you may recall, is aged between 35 and 54, and the theory is that after that we start to get a bit more relaxed. Mellow. Patient. Acquiescent. By 54 we should start to be able to suffer fools more gladly. Be a little easier to live with. Less prone to pointing out every piece of bollocks we see, wherever and whenever we see it.

Today my wife asked me what I might like as a present for my birthday.

'Nothing thanks,' I replied. 'I've got everything I want, and trying to look appreciative when opening yet another bottle of "Old Git" wine or a CD collection of songs by someone I've never heard of is a bit wearing.'

Well, I've still got a week to go. Who knows, something might happen.

8 DECEMBER

News today that someone called Grayson Perry has won the Turner Prize. There are pictures of him in the papers collecting his prize while wearing a child's party dress, and the report on BBC News said: 'In his purple party frock at Sunday's Turner ceremony, Grayson Perry seemed to revel in the fact that he was not the stereotypical cool, fashion-conscious modern artist.'

Not the stereotypical, fashion-conscious modern artist, eh? No, I think it's fair to say that collecting your prize looking like a refugee from *The Wizard of Oz* avoids that particular comparison. And the great laugh is that everyone is acting as though nothing weird is going on. Of course, it's perfectly normal for someone to collect a prize looking like Judy Garland. How urbane and sophisticated we must all be not to just piss ourselves laughing.

Now surprising as it may seem, I'm not all that grumpy about the Turner Prize. Possibly a lot of Grumpy Old Men are, but not me on this occasion. Actually, I regard the Turner Prize rather in the same way as I regard the Royal Family – not really hurting anybody and providing a good laugh once in a while. And at least in the case of the Turner Prize, we aren't picking up the tab.

The mistake that people make about the Turner Prize, and indeed about modern art generally, is to go on about it because that implies that you are taking it seriously, and that's the very last thing you should do.

Because here's the secret, and whisper it ever so softly. They aren't either.

No, the trick in dealing with all this stuff is to take on board one simple point. These people are taking the piss. They are not serious. When they decide to enter a cow turd or their own placenta for these competitions, they're just having a laugh. On you, if you let them.

What happens is that people fall into the trap of remonstrating, and then the 'artists' get the chance to talk total bollocks on the television, which is all they wanted in the first place. Because then they become a 'famous' and 'controversial' artist, and there is a long list of total air-heads with infinitely more money than brain cells who are willing to cough up squillions for a load of stuff I wouldn't exchange for a soggy piece of sashimi.

So here's the thing you need to understand: even they know that what they are saying is total rubbish.

Although it is a good laugh, even I admit that I find it a bit irritating to witness a discussion about whether a piece of film of a man swinging his penis around in all directions is 'art' or not. And another particular favourite is a close-up of an odd-looking man staring into the camera lens for 40 minutes.

But by and large you should just regard this as free entertainment. A lot of idiots talking drivel in order to con a few gullible twats. Good luck to them. So long as you don't get taken in, what harm can it do? And occasionally you'll get the odd treat of seeing a grown man go up and collect a prize while wearing a child's purple party dress.

'I don't even know who Turner was. Played for Wigan, didn't he?'

RICK WAKEMAN

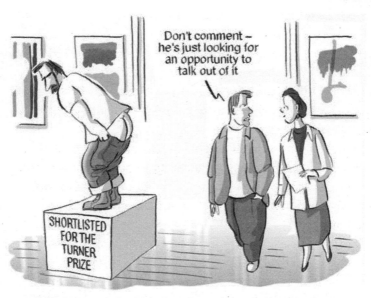

12 DECEMBER

Saw Matt at breakfast today. I only mention it because he hasn't cropped up for quite some time, and the reason is that I haven't seen him for quite some time. He's going through that phase where parents say, 'You treat this place like a hotel,' except that even I can't bring myself to say that to him because it seems like only yesterday that I was being irritated beyond endurance by my parents saying it to me. Anyway, I saw him this morning over his bowl of Cheerios. He said 'Cheerio' and made for the door.

'By the way,' he said over his shoulder as he hauled his haversack on to his back, 'remember that girl Lulu who stayed here?' I confirmed that I did. 'Saw a picture of her on the Internet. She's working as a hooker.'

Of course this does not surprise me, and I resisted the temptation to ask why he was browsing the Internet for hookers. I'm just grateful that she's not plying her trade from our guest bedroom. So far as I know.

13 DECEMBER

So today it is my birthday and yes, I'm 54.

Isn't it funny how your perspective on any particular age changes as you get closer to it?

When I was younger, if I'd ever given it a moment of thought, I would have regarded 54 as more or less dead. Possibly just a little bit short of actually smelling, but not that far off. At any rate, certainly anyone of that age could safely regard themselves as having all their best years behind them, with maybe a few years ahead in which their main task was to avoid becoming too much of a burden to the young.

Ask someone aged 25 what their definition of middle age is, and they'll probably say it starts at about 35, ends about 45 or 50, after which you enter the realm of 'aged'.

Ask the same question of someone of 38, and they'll say middle age starts at 45. Ask a 45-year-old and they may reluctantly accept that they are middle-aged, but then will quickly add, 'But I feel like a 19-year-old.' Unfortunately, as often as not, this is also a signal that they're going to start acting like one.

Pick up a magazine or turn on the telly and you are constantly hearing that people in their 50s are so much younger than they used to be

However, now that I am 54, there's no escape. Nowhere to

hide. I'm an old git. The next stop is 55 – the first respectable age for retirement. After that 60, when the best thing to do is to walk around with a bag over your head. Then 65, the traditional retirement age, and you start to think of every Christmas as possibly your last. If you are a man and you make 70 – just 16 years away in my case – you're doing pretty well.

And the big question, now that I am 54 – am I less grumpy? Remember? That's what the theory suggests, and that's part of what we set out to discover. The ages 35–54 are the grumpiest of your life, and after that you should start to get a bit more mellow.

Well, what do you think? As I enter my 55th year I'm even more utterly hacked off than ever before. With what? What with? Where would I start?

With air-head politicians who think it's OK to try to run more and more aspects of our lives, and just succeed in getting in our faces. I'm more sick to death than ever with worsening traffic, ever more fatuous television, and more and more disgusting behaviour from everyone from teenagers to tourists. I seem to have heard year in year out since I was born that crime is on the increase, that our prisons are overcrowded, that the police are under-manned (I suppose that should be 'underpersonned', but I'm also sick to death of political correctness). The NHS is in a constant state of crisis and won't ever be satisfactory because demand will always exceed supply. I hate technology, loathe shop assistants, and am sick to death of having to behave like some sort of food detective to avoid inadvertently eating something that's going to cause me an extended and painful death. Every time I see an item on the news about some food that was thought to be safe and is now known to give you some dreadful disease, I want to reach for the AK47. Every time I read a new study that a drug that everyone thought was harmless has now been found to be dangerous I want to eat my own head.

I'm entirely hacked off with waking up every day to read that we *can* do something about poverty in Africa – exactly the same stuff I've been reading and hearing since I was a small boy – yet the problems have only ever got worse.

So what do you think? Less grumpy? Yeah, right. Sorry, the thesis doesn't hold water.

'Getting old is a terrible thing, because in your head you're not ... that's another reason for the grumpiness. You actually still think of yourself as 28, and you realize that people are kinda looking at you like a sad old boy. It's bloody annoying. I hate getting old.'

SIR GERRY ROBINSON

14 DECEMBER

Sometimes it's just one thing that can set me off. Do you find that? I'll have a fairly reasonable sleep – in the case of last night it was assisted by about half a bottle of champagne left over from what passed for a birthday celebration – and then very early in the morning something will happen that will set me off for the day.

Today it was someone on the *Today* programme of all places, who reported that David Blunkett had 'turned around and said ... '

I wonder where this one originated? It strikes me that a lot of these weird expressions that don't quite make sense provided part of the soundtrack to my childhood. I remember hearing the mother of a particularly badly behaved brat on the council estate where we grew up always promising her son that 'I'll pay you', which I'm pretty confident didn't involve money. 'I'll crown you' was another one that certainly didn't seem to involve any crowns. 'Use your loaf' was a good one – I was left to deduce that 'loaf' meant 'head'. 'You'll be laughing on the other side of your face' was always guaranteed to make it even harder for me to stop laughing, with the result that the bottled-up laughter would come out in an explosion of half-eaten cheese and onion crisps, thereby getting me into even more trouble. 'Woe betide you' was another good one, sort of biblical in the dread it conjured, and was usually followed by 'when your father gets home'. Luckily, my mother had usually gone to work by the time my father got home, but I had enough sense not to ask him what 'woe betide you' meant.

Anyway, that's a diversion. The point is that I may occasionally have to hear someone in the street reporting on a strange ritualistic 'turning round' as they carry on their conversation, but if I hear on the BBC that the former home secretary has been doing it, I've had it for the morning.

'One that annoys me – "ball-park figure". You accept that; it's a ball-park, it's a rough figure. And then it occurred to me that I don't even know what a ball-park is, and if there is such a thing there's certainly not one in Britain ... I assume it's a baseball pitch or something, but even then, what's that got to do with a figure? Why can't we just say "It's roughly"?'

ARTHUR SMITH

15 DECEMBER

On the GMTV weather forecast this morning there was a warning of icy roads. 'What's caused that?' the girl with the lovely cheekbones asked rhetorically. 'Well,' she duly answered herself, 'it's the combination of the wet weather coming in and some sharply falling temperatures.' You don't say? Is that what causes icy conditions? Well, bugger me senseless. And they say that the age of public service broadcasting is dead.

16 DECEMBER

I read in the paper this morning that a 15-year study has concluded that people who eat regularly in fast-food restaurants are more likely to suffer from obesity and become diabetic. This is apparently 'one in the eye' for the fast-food lobby, who claim that their stuff is OK as part of a balanced diet. Fifteen years it's taken – they didn't say how much money – to prove something that every single person with a brain cell knows by simple observation. In fact, not even by observation – by simple common sense. Is it just me, or is this sort of thing unutterable crapulence?

17 DECEMBER

So having made a major error of judgement at Easter and on my wife's birthday, I'm certainly not going to heed her entreaties not to buy her anything for Christmas.

Encouraging her to buy something for herself that she likes seems a very sensible idea when you hear it. But when Christmas morning comes and she has obviously scoured the shops for weeks to find something I'll like, it doesn't seem such a great idea. So this year I'm determined, and tomorrow I'll break a 20-year habit, get up early and go to Kingston to try to buy some presents.

18 DECEMBER

Aaaaaargh! Aaaaaaaaargh! You recall that scene at the end of *Godfather III* when Al Pacino realizes his daughter has been mown down by bullets meant for him? The slow-motion, full-throated, primal scream? Or Donald Sutherland in the opening lakeside scene of *Don't Look Now*? Well, that's what it's been like today.

Dear God in heaven! Naturally over the years I've seen news items about crowds of shoppers, and I've heard all those 'Phew, what terrible crowds' stories from people brave enough or stupid enough to join the throng, but I've never actually experienced it. The queue to get into the Bentalls Centre when it opened looked like the crowd coming out of Wembley after the Cup Final. I didn't realize there were so many people in the whole world, let alone in one place.

I traipsed around for hours and hours and hours, browsing through perfumes, jewellery and leather goods (purses not manacles). More by way of looking for inspiration than through actual hope, I even walked through ornaments, soft furnishings and kitchen technology – but even I know better than that.

And guess what I ended up buying? Several boxes of chocolates and a perfumed candle. This evening I told her that she'll have to look for something that she likes herself. Maybe after Christmas. In the sales.

19 DECEMBER

Why do you suppose it is that everyone thinks I'm joking when I say that I don't want a Christmas tree? Every day for the last few days, my wife has asked if we can 'get the tree today', and every day I've said, 'I don't think we should have one this year.' The first few times I said it everyone laughed heartily, but recently the response has fallen more into the 'You must be joking' area.

'I'm not joking,' I say. 'We have to schlep down to the idiot grocer, pay through the nose for anything resembling a tree, scratch the car and fill it with needles as we struggle to get it home, saw the top and bottom off, put it up, it falls over a couple of times, spend hours decorating it, do a bit of ooohing and aaahing, and two weeks later take it down again.'

'Yes,' says my wife, 'it's called Christmas. Everyone else enjoys it.'

I think I remember that I used to enjoy it when the kids were young. Well, not much now I come to think of it, but I was at least willing to do it. But now that they've probably guessed that the presents left beneath the tree don't come from Santa Claus, they're almost as cynical as I am, so I just cannot see the point of going through all that hassle.

Anyway, to come to the point, when my wife finally told the kids that I really didn't plan to get a tree, the outcry left no room for negotiation – beyond my demand that they were not only present during the going up, but also during the coming down. We've all agreed we'll go and get one tomorrow.

20 DECEMBER

Needless to say, we got a tree that is far too big for the room, it fell over twice during the decoration, once when one of our idiot cats had a go at scaling it, and has already started to shed its needles. Neither Lizzie nor Matt were present for the decoration, and the wife and I were left rather sadly going through the boxes of crappy decorations that the kids had made when they were at school and which we're too sentimental and stupid to throw away.

21 DECEMBER

So last night we went to a drinks party at which someone I'd never met before talked for about 45 minutes about the new wine cellar he was having installed under his house. Marvellous process it is, apparently. Team of chaps, all Bulgarians he thought, tunnel in from outside and simply dig it out with shovels. A conveyer belt takes the soil into a skip and Bob's your uncle. Anyway, it's all damp-proofed and ready, so he's going to spend the holidays storing 5000 bottles of wine in the stacks of racks that now line the walls.

'Five thousand bottles?' someone asked him. 'Did you say 5000 bottles? The cellar must be huge.'

And you must have more money than sense, I was thinking, but didn't say.

'Yes, it's under the whole house, but only half of it is the wine cellar.' The other half, he went on to tell us, is apparently an underground sauna and solarium.

Now then, how much of a wanker do you think you have to be to tell that story at a party to people you've never met before? As regular readers know, and all grumpies will concur, ordinarily we'll do more or less anything legal to avoid these sorts of gatherings. However, on the fairly rare occasions when circumstances conspire to make us attend, I'll usually try to go to a bit of effort to keep the conversation going. But this stuff literally left me speechless.

Tonight we've got to go to another one of these sodding soirées – at Jodie and Harry's house. Jodie is an air-head and Harry is a stockbroker. Need I say more?

22 DECEMBER

Well, it turned out to be worse than even I had imagined. I'd met Jodie before, but had forgotten what a total haemorrhoid she can be. It turned out that she had been reading my last book and knew that I hated social gatherings of this sort, so she seemed to think that it was wildly amusing that we had come at all. As we had, she was determined to introduce me to everyone as the 'Grumpy Old Man'. It was exactly like that wonderful sketch in a Victoria Wood programme where they have an unemployed miner who writes angry poetry.

Having surrounded us by hapless sods, most of whom didn't know what she was talking about, Jodie begged me to 'say something grumpy', as though it was the equivalent of saying something in Czech.

'Er, fuck off?' I ventured.

Well, apparently that was the wittiest line they'd heard for several months. 'Fuck off! Did you hear that? The Grumpy Old Man said "fuck off"!'

Well, seems I've missed my vocation as a stand-up comedian. If it's as easy as that, I'm in the wrong business.

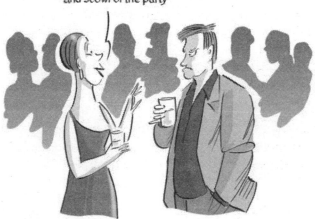

I just know you'll be the gripe and scowl of the party

25 DECEMBER

Christmas Day. Not an extended entry today because my day was just like yours. Just kind of OK.

I got some books, some CDs, some DVDs and a couple of T-shirts. Matt got a new, even more super-duper iPOD thingy to replace the one he had nicked by the hooker, and my wife gave Lizzie a load of money to buy clothes with. All really festive stuff.

And the wife's present from me? Yes, I did what so many GOMs do. I panicked yesterday and went out and bought her a pair of earrings. I was rather pleased with them, actually. Small diamonds. She did a great routine, but when she said, 'You shouldn't have,' I sensed she really meant 'You shouldn't have.'

I'll wait a few days and offer her the receipt and suggest she exchanges them for something she really wants. I know she'll agree.

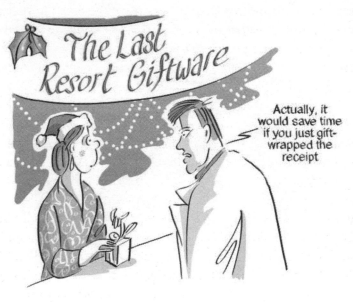

26 DECEMBER

Boxing Day. Wondered out loud, for probably the fortieth time, why it's called Boxing Day. Someone thinks that at one time we knew, but nobody can remember. Spent the day watching TV and feeling an empathy with the stuffed turkey we ate yesterday. And today. And will eat tomorrow. And the next day.

27 DECEMBER

Read in the newspaper this morning that there are protests in America against the latest reality TV series, which is entitled *Who's the Daddy?* In this show, apparently, children who have been adopted get the chance to win up to £50,000 if they can pick out their natural father from a line-up.

Now not many things that don't involve physical exercise leave me short of breath, but this makes me fear that I'm about to have a seizure. And the worse thing is, I don't know which of the participants in this circus pisses me off the most. Initially, all you can think of is that the producers of the show – guess who, the Rupert Murdoch-owned Fox network – have now reached close enough to rock bottom that they must be scraping their engorged and bloated stomachs on the coral.

But then my mind goes to the adoptive parents. Of course, I haven't seen the show, and maybe they haven't had a say, but just how anyone could stand by and allow the child they have brought up as their own learn about their real father in a reality quiz show defies comprehension and leaves me feeling nauseous. The kids themselves – I'm not sure how old they have to be – but one way or the other you have to pity them. But undoubtedly most culpable of all is the guy in the line-up who's standing there watching his real son or daughter who has never met him before identify and meet him for the first time on live television.

I'd previously thought it was a bit extraordinary to stage a dating show where the male contestants vying for the favours of the female didn't find out until the last stage that the female was a male – *The Truth about Miriam*. I'd also felt fairly squeamish when I heard about the programme in which glamorous women compete for the affections of a handsome rich bloke (*Joe Millionaire*), only to find out that he is not so much Prince Charming as Bob the Builder. However, *Who's the Daddy?* takes us into wholly new territory, where only Rupert Murdoch could lead.

Once upon a time when we heard these things we'd say, 'Well, thank God that could never happen here,' and congratulate ourselves that we as a nation had more discernment and good taste. Well, get out of here. That's what we said about all those Japanese television programmes that Clive James used to ridicule, in which contestants had to eat live maggots or have rats crawling up their trousers. We laughed our little heads off that any people could be quite so primitive and unsophisticated as to find this amusing. Well, it took about 15 years, but this last series of *I'm a Celebrity Get Me out of Here*, for my money, plumbed these new depths. And I don't know who is sicker – the contestants, the producers, or all of us for watching it.

Anyhow, watch this space. Not this year, not next year, probably not this decade, but I'll bet that *Who's the Daddy* gets here eventually. And whenever that is there'll be a fuss among the boring old farts such as myself, there'll be plenty of reservations by newspaper columnists and even politicians, but in the end no one will stop it and we'll have taken another downward step on the ladder that leads into the sewer.

And if you doubt it, ask yourself this question. If, five years ago, I'd said that in five years' time we'd be watching the alleged ex-lover of the England football captain, who sold her story to the tabloids and therefore got on to a celebrity series, jacking off a pig on live television, would you have believed me? No, and I wouldn't have believed it myself either.

28 DECEMBER

The news is, of course, dominated by coverage of the appalling devastation all around the Indian Ocean and beyond, where the latest count today is 63,000 dead. There's not much to be grumpy about in this, and all you can do is reflect on the arbitrary nature of life. One rich bloke I know left the hotel gymnasium an hour before the tidal wave struck and was saved, and the bloke who happened to be in there at the time died a horrible death. My own brother and his wife were playing golf in the hills above Phuket; had it been the morning before, they would have been on the beach. Sliding doors. We can do a certain amount to affect our destiny – mind the roads, eat sensibly, give up smoking – but in the end we are puny victims of capricious destiny.

Needless to say, grumps find much in the coverage to irritate us. For once we are not irritated by the overuse of the word 'literally' because this is a rare occasion when reporters and witnesses say 'literally' and mean it. Usually they are saying 'I was literally bowled over', when they remained upright, or 'We were literally swamped' when they had a few too many letters from viewers. On this occasion, when they say 'It felt literally like the end of the world' you know they mean it did – literally. When they say 'swamped', they mean swamped.

Every bulletin increases the number of dead – in the first few hours by tens, then by hundreds, and now by thousands each time. It was 53,000 this morning, two hours later 58,000, and when I last looked it was 63,000 – and 14 Brits. And that's another thing that's weird about coverage of this and other disasters. You always hear it, don't you – '500 killed in a plane crash but no Britons on board.' Oh, well, that's all right then, you are invited to feel; at least there were no British. It can't be anyone we know. Anyway, we already know there can't have been any Britons on board because the story is halfway down the bulletin, and it would have been the lead.

And of course there's cricket. The day after the tragedy there were three stories on BBC Radio 4 news – the tsunami, the Ukrainian elections, and the cricket. England, I believe, is playing South Africa. I just can't work out what goes through the mind of the editor who includes a report from the cricket on the day that 1.3 million and counting people have been made homeless.

My friends on GMTV this morning provided lots of coverage of the disaster, and then went to a report from Hollywood about how Anna Kournikova and Enrico Iglesias may or may not have been married. We were treated to footage of her going into the gymnasium wearing a wedding ring and apparently leaving without it. This bollocks always seems like bollocks to me in normal times, but against a background of 63,000 people dead you'd think they'd be embarrassed, wouldn't you?

30 DECEMBER

Today my wife asked me if I'd thought about making any new year's resolutions.

'New year resolutions,' I corrected her. 'If they were new year's resolutions, the resolutions would belong to the year, not to me.'

'I think I can think of one,' she said. Being smart.

Anyhow, her question caused me to reflect on how last year's resolutions have survived the 12 months. 'Must try to form a better relationship with Matt.' Well, I don't think I could honestly say I made any effort, and, in fairness, neither did he. He's 18 now, has been out on the piss just about every night since his birthday and treats me with the same healthy contempt that I showed my father at a similar age. I guess that's why they say everything that goes around …

However, my failure with Matt is totally dwarfed by my failure with Lizzie, and the only upside of the unpleasant contretemps involving her Polish friend is that he's stopped coming to the house. From what I can gather, he walks to the end of the road, sends her a text, and she goes out to meet him. I also gather he's still out of work and apparently does a bit of begging. I'm thinking of grassing him up to the immigration people. Honest.

I was also urged to try to be less impatient and to 'suffer fools gladly'. Well, on this one, to be fair to me, I did try. I clearly recall on at least two occasions trying to look interested while the air-head husband of one of my wife's air-head friends fixed me with a meaningful gaze and regaled me with their view of the growing menace from the Chinese, or their recent walking holiday in Peru. Let's face it, I failed.

I'm about 4 lb heavier than I was at this time last year, and anyone remember the CT scan? Well, that's more than the hospital did. I haven't heard a word. And do you remember the warning that in just two per cent of cases there would be numbness in the groin following an operation for a hernia? Well, see if you can guess – yes, that's right, I'm the one in 50.

And the multi-gym? Don't even go there – I know I haven't.

So what about new year resolutions this year? Should we try again? Have another go? Try to be a better person next year? I don't think so, do you?

31 DECEMBER

Well, here we are then. The end of another year. Here's me, still occasionally writing 2003 when I write the date on a cheque, and next time I look it'll be 2005. We've talked a few times through this volume about the various phrases you find yourself using as a Grumpy Old Man, which mean bugger all to anyone younger. 'Time speeds up, you know' is another of them. You hear old farts saying it and you think, 'What on earth is this sad old bastard going on about now?' Well, guess what. It does. Alarmingly.

It seems that we're going out to a 'party' at Emma and John's house tonight. I'm assured there'll be lots of people there I'll know, and that we'll have a really good time. Yeah, right.

Author's note

When, in 20 years' time, this book is part of the GCSE syllabus for Social History, it's a nice thought that swarms of bearded academics and hundreds of thousands of students will pore over every entry, every word, every nuance.

When that happens, huge and learned tomes will be written about social mores, contemporary use of expletives, disaffection and alienation, the whole caboodle.

No doubt some bright spark will persuade a gullible academic institution to fund a research project comparing the diary calendar with contemporary events, and they'll regard it as a major coup to discover that not all the stories recorded in this diary happened on or about when it says they did. This discovery will make them famous, and they'll give illustrated lectures at the RSA on how form and structure were manipulated by the author to suit his purpose. This fresh-faced twat with leather elbow patches will then posit the controversial theory that the diary might not even have begun in January and been written chronologically. In fact, it might not be a diary at all.

However, that's all for the future. It's a relief to know that no one in my lifetime would be sufficiently fucking stupid and narrow-minded as to worry or care about such a thing. Would they?

Acknowledgements

This is the bit when the author thanks his mother, his wife, his publisher, his children and his auntie for all their support; and when you read it the only thing you're thinking is – well, what else would these people do? What else is the family going to do but support the activity that's paying the bills? What else would the editor and publisher do but to publish the bloody book?

Well I hardly need say that this case is a bit different. Here we're seriously in the territory of 'above and beyond the call of duty'. Read the preceding pages and then just imagine having to share the same living space as the author. Scary huh? Think about this author's approach to everything, and then imagine what it's like to have to deal with him on the editing, organizing the cartoons, the publicity and everything else. Just ponder for a moment what it's like being the poor sods at BBC2 who have to deal with the producers of the *Grumpy Old Men* series?

I think the point must be emerging. So when I thank and apologise to my wife Marilyn, my daughter Alex; my publishers, Stuart Cooper, Sarah Reece, Stuart Biles and Shirley Patton; my commissioning editors Jo Clinton-Davis, Maxine Watson, Nicola Moody and Emma Swain; and the Controller of BBC2, Roly Keating; when I acknowledge the patience and support of all those people, I know you're really feeling for them.

And when they're reading this they're probably saying 'yeah well, it's a bit late for this now; how about being a bit nicer during the process?' But then, hey, that's tough … get over it.

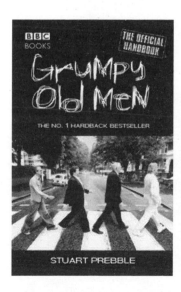
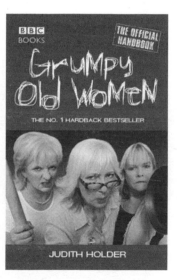